The First
and
Last
Thanksgiving

Embracing the Generations in
Our Razzle Dazzle Family

DIANNE KUBE

Publisher: Elite Online Publishing
63 East 11400 South
Suite #230
Sandy, UT 84070
info@EliteOnlinePublishing.com

ISBN-13: 978-1546484417
ISBN-10: 1546484418

DEDICATION

To Bob, My Husband

You have stood next to me and supported my many endeavors; the quiet, stable force, who manages to keep calm amidst the storms and adventures that engulf our lives.

May we always be Two For The Road!

DIANNE KUBE

CONTENTS

DIANNE KUBE

ACKNOWLEDGMENTS

To my family, friends and colleagues;

My heartfelt thanks and gratitude for your support, encouragement and love without which the story of five memorable souls may not have been told. Each of you wrapped me in courage to forge ahead to share a story that many can relate to as they face similar challenges and milestones in their daily lives. You shared your own stories of caring for loved ones and the journey you are now facing as you reach your senior years. At times you were all my guardian angels.

No words will ever match the countless acts of kindness showered upon me, I will always be eternally grateful.

FORWARD

I first put my trust in Dianne Kube twenty-three years ago when I asked her and her family, whom I had never met, to take my three-month old baby to their house from day care when I was stuck in Washington, D.C. rush-hour traffic during an ice storm. Little did I know that an endearing friendship would blossom from that initial encounter, nor that it would extend to my parents at the opposite end of the age spectrum.

There were immediate signs, however, that the Kubes would become extended family. While my infant son, Michael, sat on Bob's lap, I realized the uncanny resemblance between Bob and my husband,

Jim, and almost wondered if Michael might have been confusing them. Subsequently, the entire Kube family frequently found reasons to adopt Michael for an afternoon or evening, and when Gretchen took two-year-old Michael to visit her high school teachers after school, the two of them with their blonde, curly hair looked like big sister and baby brother. Upon the birth of our daughter the next year, Courtney immediately called Kaitlyn her own, and the families were entwined.

It did not take long for my parents to also bond with the Kubes. They often met us at Mom's and Dad's house for special occasions, or joined us for our children's activities. Mom and Dad loved people, and the Kube family's adoration of their cherished grandchildren earned them a special place in my parents' hearts. With my parents' strong educational backgrounds and professional careers, Dianne, Bob and their teenage daughters, enjoyed discussing the girls' professional goals with Mom and Dad, who, beginning their careers as professors, regarded education as an essential foundation for life.

As our friendship with the Kubes was growing stronger, my family made the difficult decision to move to Minnesota for my husband's job. I was keenly aware of the hardship our moving 1,100 miles away would place on my parents, who were already nearing their eighties. I worried not only about their sorrow from not being able to see us and missing out on so much of their grandchildren's lives, but also my inability to provide the help and support that my parents would need during their advancing years — even though they would never admit it.

Despite their zest for social activities, my parents were already experiencing some inevitable consequences of aging, and I knew that their inability to drive at night, hearing loss in my dad, and limited mobility in my mom due to arthritis would lead to lifestyle limitations and increased dependency on others. My concerns were somewhat alleviated, however, by Dianne's reassurance that she and her family would always be willing to help when needed.

Therefore, as Thanksgiving approached one year and I knew that my parents, who cherished close holiday celebrations with family, would be alone, my thoughts turned to the Kubes, anticipating that they would find room in their hearts and home for two others at their table. Thus ensued an infamous Thanksgiving gathering at Dianne's and Bob's elegant house on the Chesapeake Bay; a quiet holiday that erupted into turning their lovely home into a geriatric assisted living.

Dianne and I have shared many laughs as she recounts Gretchen's tale of her drive with four elderly folks from D.C. to the Bay, all joining a fifth senior friend at the feast, and the endearing evening that followed despite their immobility, hearing loss, and mild confusion. Then, all leaving the house utterly delighted with their containers of Thanksgiving leftovers that Dianne and Bob had graciously provided.

Two years later, my Mom and Dad realized that their large house had become too much to manage by themselves, and moved into a single-level condominium in a retirement village in a nearby community. Although I knew that it was necessary, as both of them had difficulty with the numerous stairs in the house, it was initially heartbreaking for all of us to say goodbye to our family home. I grieved for them leaving behind forty years of memories, especially of raising both of their children, playing with their grandchildren, and hosting numerous parties and bridge gatherings for their friends.

I also knew it was another acknowledgement of their progressive loss of independence. The transition was easier than expected, however, as Mom sought out every social event at the village, even turning the flu shot clinic into an opportunity for a party, and Dad remained capable to drive them to church and to social affairs with their friends. Although I remained somewhat apprehensive about the quality of their life, they reassured me that they had made the right decision.

Fairly early in my career as a physician, I was confident that I could provide solutions for my patients' illnesses. I had become adept at the medical management of chronic diseases of the elderly, knew the best specialists for treatment of more complex conditions, and could provide recommendations regarding home safety and assistive devices to improve their functionality. Consequently, I was confident that after prescribing the appropriate treatments, I would leave the patient and accompanying family member with hope that the patient's symptoms would improve and life would be easier. I also naively felt that with my medical knowledge and with my parents being generally healthy, educated, and stoic, I would not have the same challenges with Mom and Dad that burdened other families. It did not take long, however, for me to appreciate the same sense of desperation and helplessness experienced by my elderly patients and their family members.

Mom's and Dad's physical capabilities rapidly declined. Mom required hip replacement surgery, followed by double knee replacements for severe arthritis. Both of my parents' stamina and stability, along with their self-confidence diminished. I soon found myself arranging my work schedule around my husband's flight assignments as a pilot in order to have coverage for child care and the freedom to take time off to visit my parents.

Eventually, the trips back to Washington escalated to one week every month. I witnessed the challenges and frustrations that the elderly experience in performing their daily activities, of which only those who are present in the home become aware. In addition to not having the physical strength to clean the house, Mom frequently skipped showers for fear of falling. Dad spent much of the morning merely getting dressed, as he fumbled with his hearing aid batteries, buttons, belt, socks, and shoes. Due to their increasing disabilities, the effort involved in planning and fixing meals became overwhelming for them, usually resulting in a dinner of simple snacks.

My visits evolved into preparing meals for the weeks I would be gone, driving to doctors' appointments, and cleaning. I also tried to hire aides to help Mom with a shower and to provide whatever assistance they needed for a few hours each week. However, all my attempts to secure help resulted in a disaster; as soon as I returned home after arranging a service, I would receive a phone call from the agency informing me that Dad, too stubborn to admit that they needed help, refused to let the aide into the home. This precipitated a series of phone calls in which I would call Dad to plead with him to give the service a try and then call the agency ensuring them that Dad had finally agreed to their help. But, even though Dad did agree to let them in, his severe hearing loss caused misunderstandings with the aides who had heavy accents, frustrating the aides and my parents.

Most of the aides were well qualified and had good intentions. Yet, we had a few incidents that revealed this was not going to be a long term solution. There were aides who spent most of their time watching TV or on the phone, one aide invited her boyfriend to help her give Mom a bath, and another stole several hundred dollars from Dad's dresser drawer. Each event would understandably precipitate another desperate phone call from a very distraught parent, at which time I would again begin research for the caretaker who would finally provide the care I thought they needed, and alleviate the stress and guilt that constantly plagued me for not being able to provide that care myself.

The end of one's life typically involves significant emotional and physical suffering for the individual, as well as stress and sorrow for the family. The final chapter of my parents' life was no different for us, but it also provided me with new compassion and appreciation for the elderly, for whom I now hold a special place in my heart.

In mid-2010, Dad, with an apparent premonition that his life was nearing an end, wanted to make sure Mom was taken care of, so he convinced her that they needed to move to Minneapolis to be near me. The thought of them leaving the D.C. area that they called home for fifty-six years, where they maintained numerous cherished friendships and were rooted in their church, continues to break my heart. However, the inevitable day came when my sister and I accompanied Mom and Dad on the plane to Minneapolis. Then, with the help of our husbands, moved them into an apartment in a senior center.

Despite the initial warm welcome from the community, we became very discouraged two months later when we needed to move them into an attached nursing unit after Mom fell and broke her leg and Dad was hospitalized following a cardiac collapse, from which he miraculously recovered. Nonetheless, we were blessed by nurses who provided excellent care and compassion and truly respected Mom and Dad. On many visits we laughed as we watched the nurses tease Dad when he mischievously tried to get away with breaking their rules. Unfortunately, Dad passed away after another cardiac collapse only a month later, and Mom became progressively depressed, physically weak, and cognitively impaired.

Although I had the medical knowledge to work with her doctor to improve her depression and I visited her frequently, there is no medication or other treatment that can prevent the natural physical and mental decline and sense of isolation when a frail elderly person loses his or her partner in life. Unable to stay in that facility, we subsequently moved Mom into a group nursing home, where I visited her two evenings a week. I learned to celebrate those visits by coming before dinner and providing a small "happy hour" for Mom and the other residents who were able to come to the table. Just as Mom always loved a party, the residents also eagerly anticipated my visits, especially when I provided each of them with his or her choice of cocktail napkins I had brought to make the evening "festive," in Mom's words. I found that I truly enjoyed serving the residents, ensuring that they had what they needed during dinner, and felt humbled as I helped those who had lost the dexterity to feed themselves and no longer felt valued. When serving dessert, I discovered their delight in having their ice cream topped with Kahlua, and quickly learned what kinds of ice cream each resident liked, how much they would eat, and how much Kahlua to add.

Even after Mom passed away, I continued to return to the nursing home on occasion to share memories of Mom and to be blessed by the gratitude of the residents I was able to serve. I was totally unprepared for the impact that my "obligation" to spend time with Mom would have on my outlook on the end of life, as I learned to value the elderly and help them feel respected and loved no matter how debilitated they had become. I truly appreciated the opportunity to brighten their day with moments of individualized attention and simple favors.

So much has changed since I welcomed the Kubes into my life just twenty-three years ago. In contrast to being a new and inexperienced parent, I am now part of the older generation, having raised my children and accompanied my parents through the last chapter of their lives. Although I remain youthful in spirit, I've come to realize that I can no longer physically do what I could before, and pray that my children help me age gracefully and maintain my sense of humor, and that I will be able to show my appreciation for them and others.

Despite her geographical distance, Dianne has supported me through all the stages of my family's lives, celebrating the children's accomplishments, helping Mom and Dad at times when I couldn't be there, and providing support and encouragement when I felt defeated trying to deal with my aging parents, just as she did when I was overwhelmed when Michael and Kaitlyn were small children. May we all be blessed by friends like Dianne, who, by approaching life with laughter and tenderness, will undoubtedly continue to provide comic relief and reassurance as we reflect on the stories we've shared and anticipate life ahead.

Elizabeth (Engelhardt) Mandell, M.D.
In memory of Barbara and Melvin Engelhardt

PROLOGUE

Thanksgiving! It is the "All-American" holiday celebration of hope, survival, sharing and giving thanks for all our blessings. Yes, it is celebrated by all Americans; every race, religion and ethnic origin. Norman Rockwell painted its idyllic scene in his 1943 painting, "Freedom from Want;" the patriotic depiction of an American family welcoming their Thanksgiving feast. Many of us baby boomers believed in the warmth of the moment and some of us were lucky to have real life memories of joyful family gatherings. Or, at least the passing of time has transported us to remembering what ever makes us feel good.

I am a purist when it comes to the holidays, one season at a time. I do not appreciate the infringement of Christmas on my sacred Thanksgiving weekend. I refuse to decorate my abode for the arrival of Old Saint Nick on the retail calendar schedule, you know, any time after the Fourth of July! No, the crimson red and warm harvest gold that color autumn are on display for our Thanksgiving holiday and the remaining days of November as we savor the leftovers and make gallons of "Ma Ma's" homemade turkey soup.

As a child I embraced helping my mother in the kitchen as she prepared the Thanksgiving feast. My helping nature rewarded me with exclusive knowledge of making the best turkey, stuffing and turkey soup in the family. Learning and watching as Mom diced and sliced without a recipe, just many years of trial and error. My mother was not the typical 1950's - 1960's housewife. Instead, she was a 1944 college graduate who had worked at the National Archives in Washington, D.C. as an Archivist and did not know how to cook anything when she married my dad. She had always been a career woman with an avowed determination to not get married and to never have kids. Nevertheless, five children later, she turned into a full time mom and a very good cook; leaving her career behind and joining my dad in running the family business.

With matching mother/daughter aprons we shared the tasks of breaking up the bread for homemade stuffing, setting the holiday table with seasonal linen, our finest china, cut glass and crystal. My early culinary skills were launched helping Mom arrange the pimento and Roquefort stuffed crudités on the fancy divided glass platters. BUT, my favorite Mommy's helper job was inserting the toothpicks holding the cheese cubes and stuffed olives into the wooden hors d'ouvre trees; trees reserved for only special occasions. We knew it was a special holiday dinner when the trees dressed the dining room table!

Absorbing Mom's secrets has doomed and blessed me, hosting over thirty feasts in my own home with my husband and two daughters. However, our Thanksgivings have never been limited to just family. In fact, most Thanksgivings throughout the years have been shared with dear friends and all "two-legged strays" without a place to go. No one was ever turned away.

For all the wonderful memories and traditions shared over the decades, one Thanksgiving holds a special place in our hearts and in our souls. The Thanksgiving of 2004 will always be remembered for its beginnings and its endings. Retrospectively, it was a transition of time, place and generations; a time to embrace first and final visits.

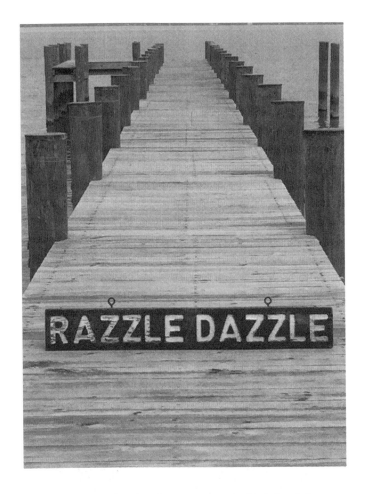

The "Razzle Dazzle" sign from my parent's ski chalet sitting on a
dock along the Chesapeake Bay.

CHAPTER ONE

IT'S STILL SUMMER

The fall of 2004 was one of the warmest I could remember in Washington, D.C., blending the seasons without a hint that autumn's waning days were looming. The past summer was a blur for my husband Bob and me as we anxiously awaited the completion of our new home being built on the Western Shore of the Chesapeake Bay. It was our mid-life crisis home; waterfront living only forty-five minutes from the District of Columbia and just what we needed to escape our supercharged Washington lifestyles. After almost two years of building delays, including a hurricane, we signed all the papers and received our keys on the last day of August. Missing our second summer on the water, we were thankful to have an "Indian Summer" to enjoy bayside living.

Over the decades, Washingtonians have migrated to the Chesapeake Bay for weekend recreation, summer vacations and to escape the cities high heat and humidity. The Bay is an estuary, a coastal body of brackish water that flows 200 miles from its head waters at the Susquehanna River to its outlet into the Atlantic Ocean. It lies inland flowing along the shores of Maryland and Virginia, the largest such waterway in the United States. Over 150 creeks, streams and rivers flow into the Bay and it is a major ecological breeding ground for birds including bald eagles, the great blue heron and ospreys. Aquatic vegetation growing in its wetlands are the nurseries for over 300 species of fish from rockfish to oysters and the blue crab.

The many varieties of fish have been a source of livelihood for generations of hard working "watermen" fishing in the bay waters. The Bay's commercial fishing industry is not run by large corporations but by local watermen, many that are descendants from British settlers who landed on its shores over 200 years ago. There are two islands located in the middle of the Bay where the English language and accent is the same dialect spoken in England two centuries before.

The watermen passed along their skills and knowledge of their trade to their children and the traditions continued.   They were so skilled at navigating the regions unique waterways that they used their mastery to design special fishing boats to harvest oysters and clams, as well as streamlined boats that enabled them to drop crab pots efficiently into the water. The watercraft are still used today and are a beautiful sight to see as they gracefully glide along the surface.

The inhabitants of the islands also created their own culinary style.   In fact, some of their recipes reached the mainland and became as famous as their history of navigation.   Smith Island takes the prize for the most well known of the cuisines with their famous "Smith Island Cake;" an eight to twelve ultra thin layer creation. Some say the recipe dates back to the 1880's when the women on the island wanted to send hearty cakes with their watermen husbands that could stand up to rough seas without refrigeration. They refined the recipes brought over from Europe and replaced delicate buttercream for a cooked icing made of fudge. This cake is so popular that in 2008 the Maryland legislature made it the official dessert of Maryland!   The yellow cake and chocolate iced original has now been joined by a variety of flavors and is always a special ending to celebrations around the region.

The Bay is also known as a sail boater's paradise with hundreds of marinas dotting its shores. Just as the watermen developed special boats for their industry, the sail boat and pleasure craft sailors also built sailing ships that are unique to navigation on the Bay.

Along with serious design, some fun traditions have developed over the years, such as the "Burning of the Socks." Once the weather warms from the winter chill and pleasure boat captains can again set sail, the tradition is to have a bonfire to toss worn winter socks into the flames and welcome in the spring.

The waterways also serve as a major shipping channel for goods coming in and going out of the United States through the commercial docks in Baltimore and the docks are host to a number of cruise ships during the cruising season.

The land use along the Bay varies from a large city, Baltimore, to the State Capital of Maryland, Annapolis, to small towns, farmland and isolated rural regions. The Bay and the villages along its shores were also strategic to the founding of our country and our defense during the Revolutionary War.

The area has a rich history of fossils from pre-historic creatures found along Calvert Cliffs, Native American settlements, maritime cultures and the United States Naval Academy; all waiting to be explored by locals and visitors alike.

My great-grandfather was the first member of my

family to venture out of the city and enjoy the beauty of the Bay. Interestingly, his discovery of the shoreline was the result of a land promotion by a local city newspaper. For every home delivery subscription, a small parcel of land was given away as a gift! His tiny lot was along the Severn River in Annapolis, near the rivers outlet into the Bay. It became my great-grandfather's refuge and therapy from his career as a designer and civil engineer in the development of buildings all across the city. He was also escaping his large extended family. My-great grandparents lived in the heart of Northwest Washington, D.C. in a large, four level, townhouse. These grand city dwellings had formal front parlors, long expansive depth to the rear of the building and many bedrooms for family and guests. The house right next to them was also owned by members of their extended family. Multiple generations living in close proximity; or, as my great-grandfather called it, one 'Razzle Dazzle Family!"

Four generations later I too was drawn to the shores of the Bay. Times have greatly changed and the days of free land are long over! The small cottages that once graced the shores as warm weather escapes from the city heat are now being replaced by full-time commuters building substantial sized homes. The local nickname given to these eclectic neighborhoods is the "Castle and Shack" communities!

My husband, Bob, also has ties to the Bay. His

father was a Commander in the United States Navy. As a Naval Aviator, he was stationed at the Patuxent River Naval Air Station for the final years of his career when Bob was in elementary and high school. The Patuxent River is one of the many bodies of water that forms the drainage basin of the Bay. Bob's childhood home until he left for college was in a waterfront community on the Patuxent River where it flowed into the Bay.

Bob spent his summer days as a lifeguard at the beach, as well as enjoying boating and swimming with his four brothers. After we met and married we would go for weekend visits to lie on the beach, boat, fish and savor many bushels of crabs on the patio of his parents' house. Bob's dad loved to fish and caught dozens of blue crabs in pots he attached to their community dock. It was a time of great abundance in the life of the Bay and special together time with Bob's family. Bob's mom loved having her new daughters in-law to hang with after raising five boys and we cherished our time with her too!

Sadly, the many attractions and commercial functions of the Bay which we all embraced have also led to changes that threatened its very existence as a habitat for wildlife. Pollution, over fishing, development and many recreational activities damaged its ecological stability. Thankfully, the efforts of private citizens, local governments and the Chesapeake Bay Foundation have begun to reverse the damage. We consider it a privilege to be protective stewards of our property along its shores. It is now our refuge, allowing us to go back to relive memories from our youthful days and it has become a place of calm from our busy lives.

Actually, "busy lives" is probably an understatement. "Extremely busy lives" may be more accurate. Having previously worked in medical administration managing community cancer centers for a number of years, my work endeavors gradually evolved and in 2004 I found myself focusing on the unprecedented changes being proposed to the American health care system. I was then serving as the Chief Administrative Officer of a national cancer organization that represented community cancer centers around the country. The position required that I spend most of my days lobbying on Capitol Hill for cancer care legislation.

The congress had already initiated sweeping changes to the Medicare laws and the field of oncology was slated to undergo major reimbursement cuts to providers. At the time, over eighty percent of all cancer patients in the United States were being treated in community cancer centers; most of the centers being privately owned by the physicians. Oncologists provided medical care and chemotherapy treatments and monitored their patients without sending them to a hospital infusion center. The community approach kept patients close to home where their families and friends could give support as well as keep the patient in a familiar environment and as close to normal routines as possible, all of which lead to better treatment outcomes. The reimbursement cuts, when initially proposed, threatened the financial viability of most oncology practices and the end result would inevitably be the permanent closing of their doors. This ultimately would lead to limiting cancer care to our elderly citizens covered under the Medicare program.

Through participating on a number of national administrative advisory boards, I had met oncology practice administrators from across the country. Upon comparing notes we collectively formed a national group to monitor legislative actions and form a lobbying team to represent the industry and save the centers from disruption. Living in the Washington, D.C. region gave me a hometown advantage to monitor the progress. I accepted the position of Chief Administrative Officer and my life took a new path. Our group hired two former members of congress as advisors and lobbyists, one Republican and one Democrat. Together with my colleagues, we began a national campaign to advise, educate and work with the key members of the committees in the house and senate that gave oversight to medical legislation. Our goal was to negotiate a reasonable solution to keep access to care available to our senior citizens and contain cost levels.

Diligently working on our endeavors in town, our evenings and weekends seemed equally busy as we unpacked to get settled at the Bay. In the midst of our frenzied life, one little distraction crept up on us without warning, the holiday season!

After a full and exhausting week of meetings, I was walking out of the Hart Senate Office Building on a sunny, November, Friday afternoon, when one of my colleagues turned to me and asked about my plans for Thanksgiving.

"Thanksgiving? We haven't given it any thought." The warm sun beat down upon my navy blue suit. After all, it was 75 degrees, who's thinking of Thanksgiving???

Harry looked at me and shook his head, "It is only two weeks away."

"Dear God! Two weeks!! What are your plans?" I asked inquisitively.

"Mandy and I are taking the kids to New York for the Macy's Thanksgiving Parade. I managed to land four tickets in the seated section on the parade route."

"Good for you! I just want to enjoy a quiet Thanksgiving weekend at the Bay. Speaking of weekends, you're going to miss your flight! We need to get you to the airport!"

I dropped Harry at National Airport and headed towards the Bay. Driving home my mind went into planning overdrive. It suddenly dawned on me that this would be our first Thanksgiving in our new home.   I need to order a turkey, call Jackie, the girls...Ugh!!!

The first call went to my youngest daughter, Courtney.   I soon discovered she was dreading the "Thanksgiving plans" call because she did not want to inform me that she had to work. This would be the first time we were not all together for a major holiday celebration. As a broadcast journalist, and being one of the newest at the network at the time, she did not have enough seniority to take off all the national holidays.

Courtney tried to let me down as gently as possible, "Mom, everyone has to work at least one major holiday this year and since I'm working on Friday and can't spend the weekend with you and Daddy, I volunteered for Thanksgiving."

I was disappointed Courtney was not going to be with us but I took comfort in the fact that she wasn't going to miss having a traditional dinner on Thanksgiving. The news bureau arranged for the full holiday fare from the best caterer in the city. Besides, now she would be off for Christmas and we would all be together!

My second call was to my oldest daughter, Gretchen. As a high school teacher she was off for the long Thanksgiving weekend and looking forward to spending the time with us and relaxing.

With a sense of anticipation in her voice,

Gretchen quizzed me, "Who else is coming Mom?" "Are Mark and Jackie coming down from Pennsylvania?"

My response was quick, "Don't know, they are next on my list to call. I will let you know what I find out."

Jackie and Mark have been our dear friends for over twenty-five years. We met when our girls and their daughter Kristen started Nursery School. Mark was a golf pro whose career took him to many regions of the country and the world. Bob and I traveled with them to Bermuda twice for events. Mark had won a number of golf tournaments on the island and developed friendships with many of the Bermudian business men. The first time we went was for New Year's to celebrate our 25th wedding anniversary and Mark's and Jackie's 27th. It was the first holiday season just three months after the September 11th attacks. Mark and Jackie were invited to go to the Mid Ocean Golf Club for the club's New Year's Eve Black Tie Gala by some of the members and they asked us to join them.

Bermuda had lost over ninety-five percent of their tourist business due to the fear of traveling as a result of the 911 tragedies. The hotels were empty and the economy had taken a devastating financial loss. Bob and I had previously visited Bermuda with our daughters. We loved the island, being warmly welcomed by the citizens and also making acquaintances.   Despite the travel concerns we decided to make the trip to support our Bermudian friends and not give in to fear.

Looking back it was a wise decision.   Mark's closest friend on the island with whom we spent much of that trip visiting became ill the next summer and passed away.   Our second trip with Mark and Jackie to Bermuda was for a memorial golf tournament in honor of Mark's dear friend.

Mark and Jackie had recently moved back to the mid-Atlantic region and we once again began to spend some of the holidays together. Once they were settled, Mark's mother, Shirley, was relocated from Florida to live near them since her health was failing and she was showing signs of dementia. So far she was able to stay in her own condo with nursing assistance. Of course, Mark's mom and nurse were welcome if she was up to the trip.

Much like me, Jackie had not given the Thanksgiving Day festivities much thought and was glad when I called. Jackie assured me that Shirley's nurses were not taking off for the holiday and she and Mark were looking forward to a night away and seeing our new home. Mark's Mom was not well enough to stay overnight and they needed a break. They would then celebrate with her when they returned over the weekend. Kristen and her husband were joining his family for the holiday in Florida.

Jackie always brought the desserts and rolls. There was an amazing bakery and farmers market in their hometown and we always managed to average one pie per person to cover all the culinary desires of those joining us. Jackie also always made her homemade sweet potato soufflé. Since it was shaping up to be just the five of us, this was going to be a relaxing, low maintenance dinner. Life at the beach!

I headed straight to my organic butcher shop to order a fresh bird, sixteen pounds should work; leftovers for all and ample bones to make gallons of turkey soup. "Miss Organization" has it all under control!

CHAPTER TWO

SLIGHT CHANGE OF PLANS

Once our daughters had graduated from college we decided to downsize our life style. The Bay house was not quite our dream home but we were happy with the builder's options. After all, it was just to be a "little cottage." Well, that plan lasted until our first meeting with the builder and design fever took hold of our brains. We went backwards from downsizing and ended up with what my husband calls "Washington on the Bay;" a traditional colonial with an air of New England. Bob and I managed to push the limits with change orders and turn a standard design into a custom home. We also took the opportunity to reupholster all of our furniture and give our traditional items a more relaxed "Bay" finish. Everything was fresh and new, even the antiques appeared revitalized. A fresh start for our new life as empty nesters had begun!

Bob's final move-in project was to clear out the half dozen boxes remaining in the garage so both of our cars would be under cover before the weather turned cold. As a Civil Engineer, Bob organized the garage better than most museum collections are stored. All the containers were labeled and neatly stacked, tools spotlessly cleaned, large items hung on the walls and small tools categorized in the tool chest drawers in a manner which would pass the inspection of any drill sergeant. It was the Saturday before Thanksgiving and all projects were completed. Our beautiful new home was ready to welcome family and friends!

Sunday morning we awoke to a bright autumn sun and beautiful blue sky. I took advantage of the crisp day and went out for a four mile walk. Solitude and a cool breeze, I was in heaven. Little did I know that our nirvana was about to implode!

Bob was out on the driveway waiting for me to return and had a funny look on his face.

"Jackie called; she seems a bit upset and needs to

talk to you. She did not go into details with me but I think something is going on with Mark's Mom."

"Okay, let me get a shower and I'll call her."

But Bob insisted, "No, I think you should call her first."

"Okay! Dear Lord, I hope Shirley is okay and not sick."

Jackie was very close to her mother-in-law and spent a great deal of time caring for her and dealing with her health issues. They tried to have Shirley live with them but the stairs in their house proved a hazard. They moved her to a one floor condo last spring and hired around the clock caregivers to fill in so Jackie, a CPA, could work during tax season. The arrangements were fine but we all knew that the next step was a nursing home.

Jackie answered the phone and sighed, "Shirley's day nurse wants to have Thanksgiving off. Her son has now decided to come for a visit and we can't tell her 'no.'"

"Jackie, not a problem! Bring Shirley with you if she is up for the trip. I know you wanted to stay overnight but not a problem."

Jackie hesitantly questioned, "Are you sure"?

"Absolutely! Does Shirley have any dietary restrictions?"

"No, we just cut her food into small portions to aid her swallowing".

"Great, it will be nice to have a member of our parents' generation with us; all will work out, and please don't worry!"

"Thanks Di."

"See you soon, bye."

All of us had been dealing with elderly parents and relatives as they adapted to living with declining health issues. Mark's Dad died in 2000 and I lost my father two years before we moved into the house. Bob's Dad was also starting to have multiple afflictions develop in the last year.

I suggested to Bob, "Now that Mark and Jackie will not be staying we need to get plenty of containers to send home leftovers. Gretchen can take 'Meals on Wheels' to Ray and Evie too!"

Bob had tossed out most of our old plastic containers when our previous home sold and we needed to move into a temporary apartment in the city as the Bay house construction was delayed. Bob was my sous-chef, dish washer and the guy who is always able to fit the leftovers into the fridge. This year we finally had a kitchen with wide open counter space, ample cabinet storage and a large capacity refrigerator.

Bob agreed, "It will be so much easier to finally have room to store the large containers; I'll stop by the local market on my way home and stock up on various sizes."

"Thanks sweetie, I will make the stock on Friday morning so Gretchen can take Ray and Evie turkey soup along with the leftovers."

My Uncle Ray and Aunt Evelyn had both been battling multiple illnesses but would not tell us when they were sick or needed assistance. Ray is my mother's little brother and her only sibling. They knew that the family was concerned for their well-being and wanted them to sell their home and move into an assisted living residence to help with their meals and medications.

Ray and Evie both had successful careers working for the federal government and never had children. My oldest brother James and his family, along with me and my family, were the only relatives living close enough to see their decline and they were not happy when we would bring up the subject of their care. Collectively, we had taken them to see lovely assisted living communities where they could have help with meals, medications and transportation but still have their privacy living in an apartment. Ray insisted it was too expensive and he became quite perturbed, so we all backed off the subject and chose to simply monitor the situation.

Over the years we shared many holidays with Uncle Ray and Aunt Evie, however, lately they declined our invitations. They were not venturing far from home and would refuse our offers for transportation. The Bay house was an hour and a half away from their residence so we knew it was not an option for them to make the trip on their own accord.

The issue of either of them driving was a big concern. Evie had always been a safe, cautious driver which normally would be good. However, the problem was driving in the Washington, D.C. region with heavy volumes of traffic and most people driving well over the speed limits, a combination that was a lethal mix for elderly drivers. Evie's careful ways became exaggerated as she aged, driving ten to twenty miles per hour under the speed limits, many times with her hazard lights flashing to slow other drivers down. Instead of being an example of responsible driving she became an obstacle frustrating other drivers caught behind her on local roads and posing a hazard on the Interstates. Driving too slow for the flow of traffic also created the potential to make her a target for road rage. Ray, we were lead to believe, was not driving at all. He had given it up when he had an accident that by some miracle had not killed both of them!

It was hard to comprehend that Ray and Evie were no longer the two people who spent a life exploring the world. Traveling was their passion.

They never traveled in first class or stayed at a five star resort, instead they chose to stay in small guest houses run by local families. As avid walkers they were the happiest strolling along the streets taking in the sights and history while blending in with the residents. They walked the Great Wall of China, climbed Machu Picchu in Peru, visited the pyramids in Egypt and the Casbahs in Morocco. In their early retirement they spent about six months of the year out of the country, wintering in Mexico and welcoming in the spring in Bermuda. Summers and autumns were spent seeing the United States or a visit to Europe.

One of their trips took them to Poland with a stop for a few days in England on the return portion. Bob and I were also traveling in Europe at the time on a business trip and, by chance, our schedules overlapped in London. My uncle and aunt were very excited to have their niece and nephew with them for one of their European adventures. They always used public transportation and Ray got a kick out of traveling on the top of a double decker bus, pointing out the sights. It was not my first trip to England so it was fun to compare our knowledge on the vast history of the city. Bob was on a tight schedule so we hired a private car to get us around between meetings; not an extravagance, it was a necessity. We invited Ray and Evie to join us in the car and we could drop them off to see area points of interest. When the car pulled up outside of our hotel and the driver got out to open the doors, I thought Ray was going to have a stroke! He turned around to Bob and asked, "What's this setting you back?"

Nowadays the distances they traveled from home were limited to taking day trips to small towns out in the mountains of western Maryland; leaving after morning rush hour, stopping for lunch at a local eatery, then heading back home ahead of the afternoon traffic congestion on the Interstates. Last October they had ventured out to see the fall foliage; the weather was dry and sunny, a perfect time to view the trees awash in color. Ray was driving after lunch because Evie wanted to enjoy the beautiful views coming over the mountains. The sun coming into the car warming the interior combined with digesting a full meal caused both of them to become sleepy. Ray slowly dosed off which resulted in the car veering off the highway and flipping over three times before coming to a stop on its side. The car was totaled. The State Police were convinced that Evie also fell asleep because their injuries were minor indicating neither had braced themselves and most likely had rolled with the car like rag dolls. Thankfully they had their seat belts on and were not ejected from the vehicle.

They were treated at the local emergency room and told the staff, when asked for contact information for their next of kin, that they could get home on their own and that they did not have any family. The investigating police officers also tried to get a name of a relative or friend to call. We were never informed about the accident until three months after the occurrence when we stopped by their home for a visit and noticed that one of their cars was not in the parking lot behind their condo. Most times we picked them up in the front of the building so we had not observed that the car was missing. We asked if it was in for service and they finally were forced to reveal the details on what had happened. I was so upset that they had not called any of us and then, to make matters worse, they kept it a secret for months!

This secretive behavior was not the first time we had been kept in the dark. Over the years they claimed that they never heard from any other relatives. We found this out by chance when my sister-in-law, Janie, and I were discussing getting her mother into an assisted living facility. I learned from that conversation that my brother and Janie had also been talking to Ray and Evie about their care and were told that they never heard from me and Bob. That is when we joined forces and kept each other informed of our efforts.

I finished my conversation with Bob about our preparatory plans, "Don't worry, if the little market doesn't have a variety of containers, I can pick some up when I do the final shopping on Tuesday. That gives us Wednesday for any last minute errands and time for me to set the table and start preparing."

No mad dashes this year!

CHAPTER THREE

THE MORE THE MERRIER

Monday was the last day I was going to do any work related activities; most of official Washington had already begun the Thanksgiving exodus traveling to cities and towns around the country. Actually, the holidays are my favorite time of year to be home. The residents reclaim their city from the hordes of tourists, elected officials and all interlopers that stake a claim on Washington for most of the year. My family has watched them come and go for seven generations and we can always rely on the knowledge that most of them will not be here forever! The locals who stay in town for Thanksgiving week and can telecommute tend to work from home on the Tuesday and Wednesday before Turkey Day or risk spending hours trapped in their cars while the gridlock of East Coast travelers passed through the Interstate 95 corridor. Bob and I planned to just battle the crowds at the local Whole Foods and Giant supermarkets.

Monday afternoon I had a surprise call from our friend Liz. She and her husband Jim had moved with their two children to Minnesota a few years prior when Jim, a pilot, was transferred by his airline. Liz grew up in Washington and was not happy about relocating to the cold climate, but it turned out to be a good move for their family. Jim spent less time commuting to his base hub airport and was around more to help with the kids. Liz, a physician, had a busy schedule and welcomed more family time together. Although, she was concerned about leaving her parents, Barbara and Melvin, alone in Bethesda since her only sister, Anne, lives in Colorado and now both would be gone.

Barbara and Mel were very involved in their church and had loads of friends. They too were getting up in years and having trouble driving at night, but they still lived in their home and had a cottage in the mountains on a lake and were not quite ready to make a move or sell either home. Liz was part of the "sandwich generation" having teenagers to keep her busy at home and elderly parents to worry about in

Washington.

"Hello Liz, what a nice surprise!"

After our friendly greetings, Liz popped the question, "I hope that I am not putting you in an awkward situation, but what are you doing for Thanksgiving?"

"I'm cooking for a small number this year; Courtney has to work so it will be just Gretchen, Jackie, Mark and his Mom."

Almost sheepishly Liz asked, "Is there any way that you can have my parents?"

"Of course," I replied without hesitation, "But I thought they were traveling out to Minneapolis to be with you?"

Liz explained, "Mom's knee is bothering her and she didn't feel up to the flight and Dad's hearing is so bad that talking to him is getting very difficult, so we decided it is a crazy time of year for them to fly on their own. We are going to wait and change their flights to come out for Christmas. Then Jim or I can fly back to Washington and accompany them on the trip."

I reassured her, "No Problem! We love your parents and it will be wonderful for them to join us once again for the holidays."

Liz seemed relieved, but then questioned, "Well

the next issue is how are they going to get there?"

I had an immediate solution, "No Problem! Gretchen can pick them up on her way out and take them back. We would have them stay the night but I don't think your Mom will be able to navigate the stairs. Bob will exchange cars with Gretchen so they don't have to climb into her Jeep Wrangler."

Liz added, "I know Bob's SUV is also high, Dad has a stool for Mom to help get her into the car."

I reassured her again, "No Problem! Gretchen will be happy to have the company for the drive."

Gretchen loves Liz's parents but she is going to kill me! Now she is not going to be able to stay.

Bob came home from the office early, toting containers from the little market down the street.

"Do they have more," I asked?

Bob asked inquisitively, "Why?"

I explained, "Barbara and Mel are now coming here for Thanksgiving. You need to go meet Gretchen tonight and exchange cars. And, by the way, she doesn't know it yet."

"Okay!" Bob responded in a supportive tone, "I'm happy that Mel and Barbara are coming out but I thought they were going to see Liz?"

"No, long story, I need to call Gretchen."

Gretchen was the reason we knew Liz, Jim and their families. While in high school Gretchen took a class in early childhood development. She was interested in pursuing a teaching career and wanted to explore what age and grade level to study. The class included visits to a local church run daycare center near our home. The students were allowed to come after school to observe and, if approved by the staff, help care for the children. Gretchen loved the babies and the center director asked her if she would like an after school job three days a week which Gretchen happily accepted.

The center accepted children from two months of age. Gretchen would come home with tales about the children and which ones were her little buddies. She even accepted baby sitting jobs from the parents on the weekends. But there was one three month old baby boy named Michael that she adored and he was all smiles when he saw her too!

Gretchen was scheduled to work one afternoon that had a weather forecast of rain and maybe some sleet in the northern suburbs. I dropped her off at the center at three while some rain was falling, but the temperatures were still above freezing so there were no concerns about the road conditions. About an hour later temperatures took an unpredicted fifteen degree drop and the rain turned into a snow, sleet and freezing rain mix, turning the road surfaces to slushy ice.

By six in the evening when the center was about to close, calls were coming in from desperate parents unable to get to the center from various parts of town because Washington roads became totally gridlocked by the dangerous road conditions. Travelers were driving less than one mile in an entire hour. Gretchen called to tell us the center wanted to send the staff home before conditions became worse but there were at lease five babies who's parents could not get there. Since we lived close by she asked if she could bring a baby home.

That was fine but we did not have any baby gear at our house. I asked if they had an extra car seat, bottles, diapers etc. Gretchen informed me they had a car seat, the parents leave extra diapers, clothes and food so we should be good. Bob was working at home that day so he and I both ventured out to pick up Gretchen and the baby. We had a four wheel drive jeep and I learned to drive on the snow and ice going to my parents mountain vacation home in Pennsylvania, so we bundled up and hit the road.

It took us thirty minutes to go two miles to the center. Once in the parking lot we discovered that the most dangerous part of our journey was walking into the building. Every surface was covered with ice. We walked in the grassy areas to try to get some traction. We were particularly nervous about taking responsibility for the baby of someone we had never met, especially in these weather conditions!

Gretchen was holding on to her precious little friend when we arrived and when we laid eyes on Michael we could see why she loved him. He was totally bald with only a wisp of blond hair visible in the light and big blue eyes. He gave us a smile and we were in love. We made the decision that I would carry Michael to the car, Bob would hold on to both of us and Gretchen would carry the diaper bag and car seat. We swaddled Michael in blankets and slowly moved to the car. He seemed to love the adventure and never cried or fussed.

Once safely home, Gretchen called Liz to tell her all was well, gave Liz our address and told her to take her time! Jim never made it back to Washington after his flights that day because the weather closed down the airports. Gretchen gave Michael a bottle, changed his diaper, and we all took turns passing him around to hold and cuddle. He sat on Bob's lap looking at the computer and smiled for a significant amount of time.

Liz arrived around eight-thirty, exhausted from the drive and anxious to see her baby. Normally the trip from her office would be about forty minutes, however, that night it took her over four hours! She walked in the front door and we all greeted her. Bob was holding Michael and the first thing she said was, "Bob looks just like my husband, Jim!" We filled her in on our evening and she told us Michael loved to sit with Jim at his computer; the little guy felt right at home! We asked her to stay the night but she reassured us that the back roads were empty and as long as she stayed off the Interstates she would be fine. That ice storm lead to a long lasting friendship!

I gave Gretchen a call to bring her up to date and, if needed, grovel a bit to get her to change her plans! Sometimes parents have moments of joy when their offspring exhibit maturity and grace. Gretchen was happy that Mel and Barbara where joining us for dinner and had no problem picking them up. She would then likely come back on Friday to do the car exchange. I suggested that possibly Courtney would come after work that same night and then both of our girls could spend the night with us since neither had done so since we moved into the Bay house. We could all enjoy leftovers, homemade soup, and some special holiday family time.

Our girls were very close in age, only a year apart; our "Irish Twins." They were also very close to each other and had invested in the Washington real estate market together when we decided to build on the Bay. At that time the girls shared a lovely home inside the Beltway. Since Bob and I were in an apartment last year, the four of us shared the previous Thanksgiving at their house.

"Mom," Gretchen thoughtfully asked, "do you think we should try to convince Ray and Evelyn to come out, I can pick them up too? I still feel bad that they wouldn't join us last year."

I agreed, "Why not? The more the merrier!"

Bob waited out rush hour and then left to meet Gretchen. I quickly called Ray and Evie announcing that Barbara and Mel were coming out for Thanksgiving.

"Please come, Gretchen will pick you up in the early afternoon so you don't need to get out of the house early."

Ray was never a morning person and as his health waned it took him even longer to get dressed and begin his day. An avid reader whose work days were spent as a researcher at the National Archives, he now spent his day in his robe, pajamas and slippers reading novels. His favorite subject matter was the American West.

They gave the usual reply, "Well, we don't want to be a bother."

I continued to prod them, "No Problem! You haven't seen our new home and it will not be Thanksgiving without you!"

Barbara and Mel spent the first Christmas after Liz moved to Minnesota with us, Ray and Evie. The two couples hit it off and I knew the fact that Barbara and Mel would be here just might entice Evie and Ray to make the effort.

Surprisingly they responded, "Yes, we will come. Thank you for having us."

As I hung up the phone I realized that I needed a bigger bird! My next call had to be to the butcher to secure a twenty-two pounder.

We were set; cars exchanged, a bigger bird ordered, and another dozen plastic containers loaded into the dishwasher to be cleaned and await Bob's leftover packing. All was well…until the phone rang at ten p.m.

"Di, its Jackie, I am worried about an issue with Mark's Mom and your new house."

"Jackie, how on earth could Mark's Mom be a problem for the house?"

Jackie explained, "We need to restrict her liquids after six p.m. because she has developed a problem with incontinence. Mark and I know how much you and Bob have worked to make your new home lovely and we would just be horrified if Shirley had an accident."

My mind quickly determined a resolution before she finished her last sentence, "No Problem! We will get plastic covers for the chairs."

Jackie thought she needed to reassure me, "She will have on Depends but sometimes if we don't change her immediately she has leaks. The problem intensifies over the course of the day and the nurses have to sometimes change her in the middle of the night if she drinks too much before bedtime. It really interrupts her sleep."

"Jackie, please don't worry, it will be fine! And there is good news, Shirley will have plenty of company her age, Barbara, Mel, Ray and Evie are all now joining us! It will be nice to have them all together. Get an extra pie!! See you Thursday. Love you!"

As I hung up the phone I turned to see Bob smiling, shaking his head. He knew from the inflection in my voice that there was an issue. I blurted out, "Where the heck am I going to get plastic chair pads???"

CHAPTER FOUR

THANKSGIVING EVE

Tuesday morning I reassess; ten for dinner, I need the extensions for the dining room table, the longer table cloth to fit the extensions and plastic pads for the furniture. After a half-dozen phone calls to home stores in the greater Washington/Baltimore area I found a Linens and Things that had six clear plastic pads to fit the dining room chairs. Hallelujah!! It is a forty-five minute drive each way but I am not taking any chances. Four hours later I arrive home, loaded down with groceries, more plastic containers, chair pads and liquor!! All is well with the world.

By Wednesday evening the table was set, flower arrangements were strategically placed around the house, the bread for the stuffing was torn into bite sized pieces and the plastic chair pads were secure. It was time to sit down to have a slice of pizza and relax. The night before Thanksgiving dinner had become as much of a tradition as watching the Macy's parade on Thanksgiving morning; pizza and a glass of wine. With all of the preparation, the last thing any of us wanted to do was make dinner.

Starting to mellow from our vino, Bob began to reflect, "It's funny, tomorrow we have ten for dinner, five elderly and five younger."

I agreed with his insightful assessment, "Yes, one on one; one for each of us to watch over. I am sure they will be fine; it's not as if we have five two-year olds coming for dinner. These are sweet, lovable elderly people."

Bob continued his thoughts on the day, "Where are we serving hors d'oeuvres"?

"Well I thought we could set them up on the kitchen table and coffee table in the family room."

Bob seemed to like my plan, then with an air of concern asked, "Do you think we should cover the couch in the family room with plastic and a sheet?"

"The dining room chairs are one thing, but I don't want to insult anyone," I quipped.

"Okay, we can decide in the morning," Bob agreed.

"Is there anymore wine?"

I never thought about the other furniture, Bob has a point, we want everyone to feel welcomed, but, if we cover the couch WE can relax.

Bob's recommendation hit a nerve, "You know, we should cover the couch. We can camouflage the plastic under a decorative throw and if it gets wet we can toss it in the wash. We can sit everyone in front of the fireplace, looking out over the water and they will be fine."

"Good, all the other chairs are wood or leather so we can just wipe them off if there is an accident," Bob suggested with confidence.

I agreed, "Yes, no problem! Oh my God, why didn't I get the stain resistant finish on the settee in the front hall?"

"Is there anymore wine?"

"By the way, the table looks beautiful."

"Thanks sweetie, I need to go to bed!!"

DIANNE KUBE

CHAPTER FIVE

THANKSGIVING DAY

It's amazing that just two short weeks prior the weather was sunny and warm, with a bright blue sky. In stark contrast, Thanksgiving morning was cloudy, grey and cold, with the wind blowing in from the Bay a bit stronger than the brisk breeze we had on Sunday. It was perfect! A great day for a fire in the fireplace with the culinary aromas filling the air, Norman Rockwell would be proud.

The beginning of the Macy's parade signaled it was the traditional time to start making the stuffing and prepare the bird. Being a germaphobe, I began to clear the counters of all decorative and kitchen items so that raw turkey meat and juice would not contaminate anything in its path. Bob was at my side ready to take orders to retrieve items from the pantry and be the one with "clean hands" when I start to stuff the bird. He had popped some refrigerated cinnamon rolls in the oven for us to graze on for breakfast and we were just about to start the cooking when the phone rang.

"Hey Dad, it's Gretchen. I don't remember the directions to Ray and Evie's, which exit do I take from 270?"

"Hi Sweetie, get on your computer and pull up MapQuest, I will go over the directions with you."

"Okay, let me call you back, bye Daddy, love you."

Overhearing Bob's end of the conversation I commented with a sense of laughter, "I can't believe that she does not remember how to get to their place! They have lived there for twenty years. Gretchen did not inherit the directions gene!!"

Bob assured me, "She will be okay, she will find it. What time are you expecting Mark and Jackie?"

"Any time after two; they are going to give Shirley lunch before they leave home and she will probably take a nap on the drive down. Gretchen should be here by two-thirty and we'll have dinner at five; plenty of time to visit before dinner and have a relaxing meal so it won't be too late for everyone's drive home."

"Good! You know I'm looking forward to seeing everyone and it feels good to know that they won't be alone today."

I agreed, "I know we wanted to have a relaxing weekend and now we really will be able to take it easy. Since no one is staying overnight, once we do the dishes it will be just the two of us and our work will be done!"

Gretchen called back for directions and to tell us she was picking up Mel and Barbara first.

"Great, just please be on time, they will all be waiting at the door looking out for you to arrive."

"Mom, relax!"

DIANNE KUBE

CHAPTER SIX

THE ARRIVALS

Gretchen called again around one o'clock to tell us that she had picked up Mel and Barbara but was still confused about the location of Ray's and Evie's building in the apartment complex. As I was attempting to explain, Gretchen interrupted, "Mom, never mind, I see them. They are sitting on the bench in the court yard." It turned out they had been out there in the cold for almost thirty minutes waiting, and Gretchen wasn't late.

Mark and Jackie arrived by one-thirty, traffic was

light and Shirley was having a good day, very alert with a big smile on her face. The outing seemed to rekindle a spark in her, reminiscent of the Shirley that always embraced being on the move. Jackie escorted Shirley into the house and immediately took her into the powder room. Mark followed carrying tote bags full of goodies from their local bakery, but he had one more item to retrieve from the trunk. Mark returned with a grin on his face and shaking his head, "We have come full circle, once again carrying a diaper bag." We both chuckled but there was also a sense of sadness.

Shirley settled in at the kitchen table to watch Jackie and I unload the pies and breads, as Bob and Mark set up the bar. Besides the usual Thanksgiving traditional fare of pumpkin pie, Jackie brought some additional favorites; apple, mincemeat, blueberry, and pecan pies in addition to cornbread, snow flake rolls, buttermilk biscuits, and cheese and pizza breads. There were also fresh picked apples, pears, a jug of apple cider, spiced nuts and chocolate covered pretzels. Add my homemade apple cake with lemon cream cheese icing to the mix and the kitchen counter looked like a page out of Southern Living's Fall/ November edition; an article entitled, "Pies, Pies, Pies and Other Goodies for the Holidays!"

Jackie sighed, "Why do we get carried away every year?"

"Because we are nut cases that want to please

everyone with their favorite foods and desserts. We never eat like this the rest of the year; it is our one excuse to have a feast. Besides, then there is more to send home with the Thanksgiving 'Meals on Wheels.'"

In reality, the cheese and pizza breads were not for today's meal, but everything else was going on the dinner and desert tables.

The house was starting to smell so good! Bob lit the logs in the fireplace and turned on the stereo for background music while I led Mark and Jackie on a quick tour of the house. Gretchen was due to arrive any minute.

Shirley seemed to be enjoying all the activity. She rarely spoke now, uttering only a few basic words, but she had a smile on her face and appeared to be comfortable. Always an active woman who was very social, she loved to shop and consistently showered her children and two grandchildren with gifts from her travels. We were all happy to see her enjoying the day.

About twenty minutes later Gretchen and her crew pulled into the driveway. Gretchen emerged rolling her eyes and quietly announced, "You owe me big!" She had a few surprises for us.

She opened the tailgate to retrieve the stool to help Barbara step out of the car and also pulled out a walker. Barbara's knee was much worse than Liz described! Our second surprise was when Evie opened her door and swung her legs out of the car. She was in a walking cast/boot. She had broken a bone in her right foot and they, of course, had neglected to inform any of us in the family that she had an accidental fall a few weeks prior. Ray seemed a bit befuddled, but otherwise fine and Mel was his usual delightful self.

With only two steps to navigate on the front porch and one into the house, we lined the front walkway, porch and entrance hall like a fire bucket brigade to safely assist our fragile guests. Once inside a chorus of "Oh so lovely," "It is beautiful," "Oh my little niece must be loaded," "Can we have a tour?" started with all talking at once.

"Thank you! Let's get your coats off and get settled then we would love to show you around." I helped Barbara navigate her walker down the hall and into the family room where she announced that she had found her spot to sit! She proclaimed emphatically, "Oh, here's my seat, Mel, I'm sitting on the couch!"

Barbara was adorable. She stood about 4 feet 11 inches and was almost as wide due to her shrinking stature from osteoporosis. She also loved to talk and she managed to narrate everything that was happening at any given moment. A devoted mother and grandmother who had a career as a college Professor, teaching French, she was a true lady that followed all the proper manner of decorum and etiquette. She just loved to chatter!

Mel was tall, well dressed, and courtly in manner. He had a Doctorate in Education and also taught at Universities. They moved to Washington, D.C. when Liz and her sister were babies and Mel headed up specialized education programs for a number of Federal Government agencies. He was also a sweetheart, a distinguished gentleman and so kind, but he couldn't hear anything spoken in normal tones. We always laughed that the more Barbara spoke, the more Mel's hearing seemed to decline. Nature taking care of its own!

They may have slowed down but they still loved to keep some of the traditions of their generation, having a cocktail hour before dinner, discussing their day and reminiscing about their family and the wonderful times spent together. At any moment it seemed Bogie and Bacall would enter the room and join in the fun; another era sadly slipping away.

CHAPTER SEVEN

THE TOUR

On quick assessment; two can't walk, one can't talk, one can't hear, one is a bit confused and one never stops talking. This combination will surely make for a Razzle Dazzle Thanksgiving! With Barbara and Shirley happily perched in the great room, Ray, Evie and Mel wanted to explore the house. Mel would be fine on the stairs but Evie and Ray were an issue. Our stairs were a bit daunting for even the able bodied; they rose more than the average staircase due to the high ceilings and curved halfway up. Bob led the way and two of us took up the rear to catch anyone losing their footing. We managed to navigate without any stumbles and they loved exploring a new habitat.

Every door was opened to see the size of the closets and they counted the number of sinks and toilets. They stopped at every window to discuss which had the best view of the water and my uncle loved to point out that the rolled pillows on the bed were French! Actually, I had them made by a local seamstress, "fancy neck pillows." I am sure he saw rolled pillows in Paris and assumed that these had to be a product produced by the French. I smiled and told him he was correct.

Ray could have afforded to live in a single family home but could not deal with the emotional burden of the cost and upkeep. He was more than thrifty, he was downright cheap!! He and Evie had bought a lovely home in a Washington bedroom community thirty years ago and he acted like he had moved to the wilderness. My grandparents were still alive at the time and they would all go to the "country" for the weekend.

Ray was not domestic nor had any talents with tools or machines. A lawn mower to him was equivalent to running the space shuttle and if anything broke it was as if a natural disaster had taken place. They kept that house for less than a year and he was extremely happy to get back to their little one bedroom apartment in the city. They stayed there until retirement and then bought a two-bedroom condo eight miles outside the Beltway, which was the maximum distance he would allow himself to move from his beloved city. For a couple who traveled the world and who loved the wide open spaces of the great western plains, they did not want to live anywhere but in the comfortable surroundings of their hometown city of Washington, D.C.

This crowd had lived during the depression, wars, the space age and substantial growth and development. It was amazing to see how their personalities had been influenced by those years and the impact on living their lives; frugal, spendthrift, world traveler, homebody, adventurer, creature of habit, well read, successful, generous, self-deprecation or not worthy of having anything! Any and all terms could describe them and how they viewed themselves. All of which made spending Thanksgiving with these five wonderful people so special; they gave thanks for all they had every day. Time and declining health was catching up with their bodies and minds but in their eyes they were still young and eager to celebrate.

Once back on the ground floor the party started to come to life, cocktails flowed and we brought out the hors d' oeuvres. After seeing how frail our five special guests appeared, I decided to place all the hors d' oeuvres on the kitchen table so they could all sit together and enjoy each other's company and it would be easier for them to reach the food.

That decision turned out to be wiser than I could

have anticipated, depth perception and unsteady hands proved to be a challenge. Evie sat next to Shirley and helped her with selections to add to her plate, Barbara examined all the items giving everyone a verbal detailed description, and Ray and Mel ignored the ladies and dug in by loading their plates with shrimp and savoring the treats, not saying a word. Thankfully our kitchen, breakfast room and family room are an open concept design, really one big great room, so we could keep an eye on everyone and help if needed.

Evelyn was the spryest of the three ladies and did not allow her broken foot to slow her down. But in reality she had the most fragile health conditions of them all. She had brittle juvenile diabetes and had suffered many side effects of the disease over the years. Evie had dozens of incidents that left her hospitalized including falling into a number of diabetic comas. She had falls that resulted in two broken hips and the diabetes had caused nerve damage in her feet. It was a miracle she still had her eye sight. I always worried about her vision! A dear friend described going blind as the eclipse in one's life and I prayed that Aunt Evie would never face that challenge.

Evie grew up in North Carolina and still had a sweet southern accent, unassuming and always a lady. No one would ever guess that she had been an eyewitness to history. She served as an executive assistant at the American Embassy in Paris and was stationed at the White House for over twenty years, serving from the Kennedy Administration to the Carter Administration. She was an assistant to Secretary of State, Henry Kissinger and was one of a handful of people that was privy to the efforts leading to the China Peace Talks during the Nixon administration. A chameleon who could keep secrets!

CHAPTER EIGHT

BREAKING BREAD

The dinner was starting to come together; the bird was out of the oven and the stuffing was removed. It was time to finish making the vegetables, mash the potatoes and whip up the gravy. I was joined by my four helpers behind the kitchen center island; Bob, Gretchen, Mark and Jackie were lined up awaiting my direction while Gretchen filled us in on her earlier hour and a half drive which had us all giggling.

Mel was her co-pilot sitting in the front passenger seat commenting on her outstanding driving abilities on the Interstates. Ray told her that girls should not be driving alone on the highways, it was too dangerous. Evelyn just smiled, enjoying the ride and scenery as Barbara narrated all she saw along the way.

Mark, always the one with the dry wit, was cracking jokes and teasing Gretchen.

"Just think Gretchen, you get to repeat the ride and the conversation on the way back!"

"Great!!!" Gretchen responded with more than a hint of sarcasm, "Ray will want someone to ride shotgun since it will be dark and a **girl** will be driving on the Beltway." She was quick to add, "You guys owe me big!!"

Jackie just stood shaking her head and repeating the same statement, "Let's go out next year!!"

Bob was waiting for directions. "Ok, what is the game plan and seating order?"

That was my cue to begin assigning responsibilities to my "kitchen crew." "Alright, let's get started! Before we move everyone in to be seated, Gretchen please fill the water glasses, Mark light the candles and open up a bottle of white and a bottle of red wine, Bob you can start to carve the bird, and Jackie and I will finish the veggies."

We were a fine tuned machine, veterans of years of shared celebrations. Jackie leading the team at her home and me leading us here, the guys happy to help and glad they did not have to be responsible for any decisions. This level of precision evolved from humble roots, many of our long past Thanksgivings were not very grand in design or location, nor did the preparations always go smoothly.

Our first effort at cooking a turkey was when Gretchen was only four months old. We could not travel to visit either of our extended families because Bob had to work the Friday after Thanksgiving. We were living in a small two bedroom walk-up apartment with a shoe box kitchen, no counter space, no dishwasher and a tiny oven. Needless to say we cooked a tiny turkey that year! I managed to have enough stove top burners to cook the corn, green beans and mashed potatoes with a spare to make the gravy. No homemade rolls, Pillsbury provided their crescent creations, and no sweet potatoes or desserts were on the menu. The table was set with our white everyday dishes and stainless steel flatware. Although it was a basic beginning, we were proud of our accomplishment to make a meal and lay the foundation for our own family traditions.

Over the years we have had the usual spills, power outages, bad weather, backed up kitchen sink and burnt rolls. All these mishaps served to strengthen our fortitude to not "flip out" as procedures went awry and, instead, we learned to a take a deep breath and solider-on! This included the year I bought a frozen turkey. We awoke on

Thanksgiving morning to discover that it had not totally defrosted. Actually it was still frozen solid except for the legs and wings. We went to plan B and quickly sanitized the bathtub, filling it with lukewarm water to immerse the bird to try to hasten a warm up! Once the bath water turned cold we drained the tub and refilled it with tepid water repeating the scenario until the turkey was a temperature ready to prepare. Yes, it was the first and last time I ever purchased a frozen bird!

With the lessons of past years behind us, our "Thanksgiving Team" was well prepared to execute today's celebration with precision. Ten place settings with four seats on each long side of the dining room table were set. The newly purchased plastic pads were on six of the side chairs strategically positioned for our special guests. We decided that Jackie, Gretchen and I needed to be seated nearest the kitchen door and that the two special guest couples should be in the four seats on the far side of the table, with Shirley next to us on the far end so Jackie could monitor her portions and liquids. The extra chair pad was on the seat next to Shirley in case she spills or drops any items. Bob and Mark would sit at each end of the table. The plan was ready for action!

Bob announced it was time to move into the dining room to be seated and all five positioned at the kitchen table attempted to move at the same time which is when we noticed that they all were covered with crackers, bread crumbs with drops of crab dip and cheese clinging to their clothes and covering the new hardwood floors. They all had plates and napkins but balancing canapés and gooey dips on crackers and bread was more of a challenge for them than we expected.

"Let us help you to your seats!!"

Mark with a Cheshire cat grin on his face whispered, "Don't you now wish you had a dog Di?"

"Oh god!!! Don't worry, we will clean it up!!" I'm just glad we decided to forgo a rug under the kitchen table.

Bob looked at me, "What about the dining room?"

"Okay, they will have large linen napkins and we need to help push the chairs in as close to the table as possible so they can reach. It will be fine!! I hope!!"

One by one we each took an arm and escorted the gang of five to their seats. Barbara once again provided running commentary and shrieked when she saw the table set with holiday finery of china and crystal in autumnal colors.

"Oh Dianne, your table looks beautiful!!!"

This was her first viewing of the living and dining rooms since she did not take the tour.

She added, "I always say that every bride needs a

ary doryr

good set of Lenox!"

"Thank you Barbara, it is my pleasure, I too love to have a properly set table and it's so fun to take out my seasonal pieces."

Our cherished guests all beamed and felt so special!

Of course I was far from being a bride and never a fan of Lenox, except for their Christmas patterns. Bob and I had eloped so we never had a gift registry. It actually took years of scavenging through consignment shops, antique fairs and department store sales to amass my collections of china, fancy cut glass and crystal. Truth be told, I was known as the "Princess" of china and glass. It transported me back to having tea parties as a little girl and setting my mom's holiday table, a passion shared with my dear friend Sally, known as the "Queen" of china and glass.

Sally and I had met when chaperoning a dance at our children's high school and instantly formed a bond. Turns out her Mom was a member of the Washington Glass Club and she had been studying the history of china and glass patterns for years. I inherited some of my Grandmother's pieces and finally met a kindred soul who also had special pieces from the Washington region. Together we had not only traveled around the United States in our quest to build up our treasures, but Sally served as an

American Diplomat in Europe so we hunted the back roads of Hungry, Austria, England and Italy together. Mark always said that I needed a red velvet rope to keep everyone out of my "pretty rooms!!"

With everyone seated and the serving dishes filled to the brim it was time to say grace. Gretchen, being the youngest, led us in prayer. Evelyn closed her eyes and Ray fidgeted in his seat, Mel and Barbara folded their hands together, and Shirley smiled.

"Bless us oh Lord and these our gifts for which we are about to receive, and give us this day our daily bread, in Christ our Lord, Amen."

I asked if anyone had anything that they wished to add. Mel, a devoted elder in his church, spoke up and said, "I too wish to give thanks to God and I want to say thank you for having us to this wonderful feast and welcoming us into your new home. We are so blessed to be here." Barbara added, "Amen to that!"

Evie giggled and Ray chuckled with nervous laughter. Ray, though being raised by the son of a Methodist minister and educated at parochial schools, was not known as a church going gentleman. But he was a big fan of any good meal and the sights and aromas were too much for him to sit and be social and pious, he wanted to eat!

"That was lovely Mel," I said supportively. "Thank you for the kind words. We are so happy to have you all join us and be together to share our first Thanksgiving at the Bay. Okay, let's start serving."

Bob, Jackie, Mark, Gretchen and I sprang up from our seats to assist with fixing plates. We each grabbed a serving dish and started around the table placing the bounty close to the dinner plates and within easy reach of frail hands. Barbara was announcing the contents of the platters and bowls proclaiming, "Oh it all smells so good," as each item passed by her plate. As the china dishes filled to almost overflow, Jackie cut Shirley's food into bite-sized pieces and gave her a small glass of water. Mark served the wine. Once the "gang of five" were set, the five members of the "wait staff" served themselves and Bob offered a toast.

"To many more happy holidays and celebrations together. Thank you all for coming and making this a very special day! CHEERS! Let's eat!"

Not another word was uttered as we all savored the feast and took in the ambiance of the moment. Eventually small talk and fun chatter began to go around the table causing laughter and plenty of smiles. The "gang of five" all appeared to look ten years younger in the candlelight and the companionship rekindled their energy. After everyone cleaned their plates and a few minutes of rest passed we offered seconds.

The ladies declined but all the men were happy

to help themselves to another round, though much smaller than the first helpings. I went into the kitchen to refill the gravy boat and start the coffee and tea for dessert with Bob right on my heels.

"I am fine sweetie, you go back to the table, we will clear after you guys finish."

With a great deal of concern in his voice Bob said, "I need to talk to you!"

I responded with equal concern, "What's wrong?"

He continued, "Is there something else you're not telling me about Mark's Mom?"

"No, what's going on?"

"Mark's mom is hitting on me!!!"

"What!?"

"Yes, she keeps leaning over and grabbing my legs under the table while smiling and blowing me kisses!!"

"For God sake!! Get a grip, she has dementia, she doesn't know what she is doing!!"

"Well, you know what a flirt Mark is; after all she is his mother."

At this point Jackie and Mark came into the kitchen to check on us.

Without hesitation I immediately announced "Mark, your mother is hitting on Bob."

Mark and Jackie burst out in laughter. Mark said, "Yes, she throws kisses and gets all excited when the male physical therapist visits her too."

"She is grabbing Bob under the table," I added.

"Oh Bob, she just thinks you're cute," Mark teased.

Bob was not amused. Gretchen then joined us and announced, "Shirley is drinking from everyone's glass."

Jackie threw up her arms and proclaimed, "Oh no! She won't make it home without an accident!"

Jackie bolted back into the dining room.

I tried to calm Bob's concern. "Okay, let's all sit down and enjoy the rest of the meal. Bob, just ignore her!"

Bob shot back "Now we know where Mark inherited his flirtatious wit!"

Poor Bob, he has such respect for the elderly and it appeared his first "Mrs. Robinson" moment was about to unglue him.

We managed to get through the remainder of the meal without Bob suffering any physical harm and all liquids were removed from Shirley's reach. Ray excused himself to go to the powder room after a gallant second helping. It was time to set up for dessert.

We cleared the dishes and retrieved the warming pies from the oven. Clean dessert plates, cups and saucers were passed. Gretchen grabbed the freshly whipped cream from the refrigerator and ice cream from the freezer. The cake and pies filled the table and sideboard along with the candied pretzels, nuts and fruit. Yes, one desert per person, the tradition continues.

Evelyn beamed, she loved sweets even though it was not good for her health. Her diabetes caused cravings for candy and cakes. I checked with Jackie and Gretchen to see if they had noticed if Evelyn had taken her insulin. Evelyn was so careful with her medications but with all the excitement I just wanted to double check. Gretchen said she saw her go into the powder room with a small blue cosmetic bag just before dinner.

"Good, that is her insulin bag. I just don't want anyone to have any health issues tonight."

"Speaking of the powder room, has anyone seen Ray?"

Bob left to check on him and found the powder room door opened and the room empty. Ray wasn't in the kitchen or the great room, so Bob headed to the front of the house. That is where he found Ray, standing in the Library looking lost.

"Ray, are you okay?"

Seeming somewhat confused, Ray responded, "Yeah, you know, this house is so big I was not sure which way to go when I came out of the bathroom. You Know, You Know!"

Ray had a nervous laugh and repeated the words "You Know" when he became anxious. He was a bit embarrassed but also seemed amused with himself. The house is not that big; we knew it was another sign of his decline and sundowners confusion. Bob led him back to his seat and did not say a word, just smiled and patted Ray on the back. All was forgotten as soon as Ray's eyes took in the array of desserts set out before him on the table.

The pies were sliced, the cake cut and served, fruit and nuts passed. The tea and coffee flowed from the silver service into the fall patterned china cups. I had mixed orange colored sugar used for decorating cookies with the white granulated in the sugar bowl to add a festive touch. Barbara noticed every little nuance of the decorations, from the crystal turkey candle sticks and salt and pepper shakers to the amber water glasses. It was so fun to see the delight in her eyes as she took a sip of her tea with the special sugar. "Oh, real whipped cream too!" Barbara proclaimed as she sampled the pumpkin and apple pies. It made all of us feel so special to put forth the effort to have an all-American traditional holiday meal and to make the ambiance of the setting just as special.

As everyone finished their dessert and took seconds we decided it was time to start packing up the leftovers and begin to wind down the evening. Our guests had more than an hour of driving time ahead of them and we noticed that the wind had picked up and the temperature was dropping fast. There was a chance of light showers, with the wind howling and the leaves falling on the streets, it could become slick on the road surfaces. Uncle Ray would be a wreck with his grandniece at the wheel if it started to rain.

Everyone, young and old, offered to clear the table and help with the dishes. We thanked everyone for their offer but insisted that Bob and I had the whole evening to load the dishwasher and do the cleanup. The Budapest crystal glasses that I had hand carried from Hungry survived international travel, but I wasn't sure they could survive the frail grip of our special guests.

CHAPTER NINE

THE DEPARTURES

We encouraged everyone to take a bathroom break so they would have a comfortable ride on the way home. Jackie took Shirley into the powder room to get her ready for the trip back to Pennsylvania.

Bob lined the kitchen counters with the plastic containers and began packing them with turkey, stuffing, mashed potatoes, veggies and gravy. I took note of everyone's favorite dessert selection and packed containers with the cake and pies. We gave everyone a container with a heaping serving of whipped cream and we packed rolls into aluminum foil for easy reheating.

Bob even gathered sturdy shopping bags with handles to transport the containers. We made sure that everyone had enough food to take care of their dinner needs for the rest of the weekend. I added holiday napkins, cocktail and dinner size, and made sure that Barbara had the holiday sugar for her coffee and tea. The Meals on Wheels were ready for the road!

The "gang of five" sat in front of the fire while Mark and Jackie loaded their car and Gretchen and I searched the house for everyone's belongings so not to leave house keys, wallets or purses behind. Bob retrieved coats and hats from the front hall closet and lined the shopping bags filled with goodies by the front door.

I could see that all five were starting to get heavy eyes, it had been a big day and they had a big meal. We decided to help Gretchen load up first before Mark and Jackie headed home.

I opened the front door to check on the weather and it immediately blew inward as if a tornado was sweeping through. The smaller trees were bent over and leaves were swirling in the wind. The mums I had arranged in baskets sitting next to the pumpkins on the front porch had blown over. It became evident it was going to be a challenge loading everyone into the cars with gale force winds. Bob heard the door bang and came out to check on me.

"The wind is wild! We need to have one of us on either side of our special guests to help get everyone safely into the car. Let's start getting coats on and move them out one at a time."

We moved Gretchen's four passengers to the front entrance hall to begin the goodbyes. Hugs and kisses were being given all around and many kind words of thanks were expressed for hosting the dinner. We also expressed our appreciation to everyone for joining us for our first Thanksgiving party at the Bay.

I wrapped scarves around Evie and Barbara and told everyone to hold on to their hats! Melvin insisted on carrying the food bags to the car. He actually was fine helping and was good at assisting with Barbara. Ray tried to grab one too but he was not sure footed so Gretchen asked him to carry Evelyn's smaller purse to the car so he felt useful.

Gretchen ran ahead to start the SUV so that it would be warm inside as we escorted the first two, Barbara and Melvin. Barbara's coat was caught by a wind gust and it flew up in the back and almost went over her head; she was greatly amused and giggled. Bob and Mark steadied her on the stool and into the back of the vehicle. Once Barbara was settled into the middle of the back seat, Mel and Gretchen placed the walker, stool and Meals on Wheels into the tail section.

We then headed back in to retrieve Ray and Evie and caught them attempting to come out on their own. Our front porch is made up of slabs of decorative stone and the last thing we needed was a fall. Bob and I ran up and took their arms to get them down the steps.

"We're fine," Evie insisted.

I told her that the wind was so strong we did not want them to trip or drop their belongings. We walked them to the car and got them settled. Gretchen gave us hugs and loves and we wished her good luck for her journey. As she pulled out, her precious passengers waved and threw kisses until we were all out of sight.

Mark finished loading up his BMW sedan with their share of food and treats for the weekend and Jackie and Bob led Shirley to the car. I took one last trip around the house to check for any remaining items.

When Shirley sat down in the back seat she turned and smiled, then uttered her first words of the evening, "I'm leaking, I'm leaking!" Mark and Jackie looked as if they were about to cry! Mark had towels down and plastic on the seat so they decided to just hit the road since Jackie had just changed Shirley's Depends. The wind was getting fiercer, and they were heading north to colder temperatures. Our fear was that the looming rain showers could turn their roads into black ice.

We thanked them for all their help and contributions to the meal then gave hugs and kisses all around once again. Jackie was concerned that we were left with the cleanup, but we assured her that it was not a problem. As they were getting into the car Shirley began to blow kisses to Bob and winked at him. Bob smiled, winked and blew her a kiss back. Shirley shrieked with delight! At that point the four of us lost our composure, we laughed so hard we began to cry. Shirley indeed had a wonderful Thanksgiving!

DIANNE KUBE

CHAPTER TEN

THE CLEAN UP

Bob and I watched as the tail lights of the Beamer faded into the distance and then walked back into the house to assess the damage. We pushed the front door closed against the wind and secured the lock. We turned around to find our lovely home had been turned upside down. I guess we did have five two-year olds visiting!

In addition to the stacks of china dishes and crystal to be hand washed, furniture had been moved around to accommodate additional seating and the movement of Barbara's walker. Breakable items had been placed away from heavy traffic areas and the potential to be knocked over, the kitchen floor was thick with dropped food and a mountain of pots and pans sat on the stove.

We decided to roll up our sleeves and pull an all-nighter if needed to put the house back to pre-Thanksgiving condition. Bob started to clean off the counters and load the dishwasher as I got on my hands and knees and started to scrape cheese and dips off the floor under the kitchen table. Thankfully with all hardwood floors around the house and only a few decorative carpets I could wet Swiffer the majority of the floors and vacuum the remaining surfaces. I washed down the kitchen table and took off all the protective coverings on the couch and chairs.

After the dining room table and sideboard were cleared and the table linens were placed into the washing machine we removed the table extensions and reset the room back to everyday living. Three hours later as we dried the last crystal goblet, packed the silver flatware into the silver box and finished loading the second set of dishes into the dishwasher, we began to see our home re-emerge from the chaos.

Jackie called to tell us that they were safely home and that Shirley fell asleep less than five miles from our house. Her night nurse was on duty when they arrived and helped Jackie get Shirley changed and settled into bed. Jackie told me at a later time that

Shirley slept most of the next day, she had partied herself into exhaustion.

Gretchen also checked in to say she was home and her passengers delivered to their doors. She drove Ray and Evie home first to avoid Ray being upset as she pulled away alone in the car. He did not approve of girls driving on the Interstate and they should never drive anywhere alone at night!

She said that the tryptophan from the turkey set in and three of her four passengers fell sound asleep before she reached the main highway. The only one awake was Barbara who kept Gretchen company and relived the day moment by moment. The only other noise was the chorus of snores from the three sleeping beauties.

Gretchen walked Ray and Evelyn to the front door of their building and attempted to walk them up the flight of stairs to their condo, however, they insisted on standing at the front door to watch her leave the complex. They waved goodbye and watched her drive off into the night.

It was not until many months later that we learned Ray turned to go up the stairs, lost his balance and fell on his knees. He was trying to help Evie up the stairs while holding on to their bag of food and treats. He had abrasions and cuts on both knees and legs, it was a blessing that he did not break both knees. By some miracle Evie managed to stay upright when he fell and he saved the bag of food! The Meals on Wheels stayed intact, not a drop spilled!

Finally, the cleanup was complete! We decided to take showers and get comfortable, then come down to watch the fires waning flames and have a Baileys for a nightcap. Bob and I did not have time for cocktails or wine earlier because we had too much to do and did not want to get tired. Actually, no one had more than one or two drinks over the course of the afternoon and evening. Driving and age played a role in keeping everyone under control. The days of over doing it at the holidays are far behind all of us!

It was now our turn to relax. Bob looked at me and sighed, "I never knew how lucky I was to have such healthy parents. Dad has some minor medical issues and has slowed down but look how active he has been until just the last few months; fishing, golfing and working on projects around the house. Both of my parents still enjoy swimming in their pool and gardening. My mom is really amazing, she would have been right in the middle of the cooking and the clean-up. She takes impeccable care of their house, runs all over town in her sporty car, babysits and they are both older than Ray and Evie."

I nodded in agreement, "Your parents are both what we all aspire to be in our 80's. They have always been active and are young in sprit too! It is intriguing to me to see how people age. It must be a combination of lifestyle, attitude, genes and good luck thrown in to keep living and not just existing. I wonder if any of our five special guests will ever visit us again here at the Bay."

"I am grateful that they all managed to come out today. Maybe Barbara and Mel will come out with Jim and Liz when they are in town."

"Yes, maybe."

DIANNE KUBE

CHAPTER ELEVEN

THE DAYS AND YEARS ROLL ON

Eight months after Shirley shrieked with delight at the attention of a blowing kiss and a wink she totally stopped talking and walking. Mark and Jackie reluctantly moved her to a nursing home. Even with around the clock nursing care the pitfalls of being in a skilled nursing facility took their toll. Shirley developed a bedsore which led to a MRSA infection and in less than eighteen months she was the first of the gang of five to depart.

Barbara wrote me a lovely thank you note

recounting all aspects of Thanksgiving day. She wrote like she talked, filling every space on the card, even writing upside down to make a point and to not leave any unused paper. I saved it to give to her granddaughter Kaitlyn, our godchild, as a delightful memory of her grandmother. We often teased that Barbara loved to chat, but she was also a good listener and kept her spirits high no matter what challenges she faced.

Mel and Barbara finally decided to sell their two homes and move into a lovely condo in 2006. We all decided to make one last trip to visit their lake house before the new owners took possession. Over the years our families spent many summers together vacationing on the lake, boating and swimming and we all loved to go to the Harvest Festival weekend every October which managed to fall on or around my birthday or Michael's birthday which were a day apart. Traditionally that was the weekend Jim and Bob would take the boat to the marina for winter storage and pull the floating dock onto the land. The current floating dock was built by Jim and Bob as a thank you to Barb and Mel for hosting us at their home. The lake would freeze in winter and the floating docks were preferred by the residents because they would last longer. That ritual signaled the closing down of the lake house for the season, but this time, sadly, it was our last time to close up the house and say goodbye.

The move proved good for them for a few years. They managed on their own another four years until Mel started to develop cardiac disease. Liz then decided to move them to Minnesota. Liz and I packed up Barbara's Lenox and crystal, the condo was sold and they moved into an assisted living facility a few miles from Liz's and Jim's home. Four months after the move Mel went into cardiac arrest and died. He never lost his elegant style and was mobile and brilliant until the end. He had been the healthiest at Thanksgiving so we never expected him to be the second of the "gang of five" to leave us.

Ray and Evie continued to have mounting health issues and were becoming increasingly fragile. Ray, always a lovable teddy bear, started to get agitated and paranoid. He would make phone calls to us at all hours of the day and night claiming that the banks were stealing his money. When Bob and I would leave town he would make calls to Courtney at work telling wild tales that someone was selling his stocks and bonds and taking money from his accounts. He trusted her because he thought she must be smart since she was in the "news business!" His health was rapidly declining and he was having mini-strokes. Neither of them were eating properly, their hygiene habits were almost nil and the condo was not being cleaned.

Evelyn's blood sugar started to fluctuate to dangerous levels because her nutrition was so poor and her medications were no longer able to control the levels consistently. She was having blackouts and collapsing every few months. There was one incident that will go down in family lore for the absurdity of the moments surrounding the event.

Evie passed out and fell onto the floor of their bedroom. Fortunately, Ray had enough awareness to call for help. The only problem was that he did not dial 911 but called a private number. The young man who answered the phone thankfully realized that he had an elderly, confused man looking for help. He asked Ray for his address and Ray gave him an address but not his own; he gave our Bay house address! We later learned that Ray was trying to call me and not 911. He dialed the wrong number but somehow knew my address!

I had just arrived home from a long day working on Capitol Hill. Bob was out of town on business and I was looking forward to taking a relaxing shower, getting in my pajamas, and having a quiet evening. Just as I closed the garage door and put down my purse, I heard a siren off in the distance. A few minutes later an ambulance pulls into my driveway and fire/rescue personnel rang our doorbell. At the time our local engine company was in their annual fundraising drive and Bob had written a donation check before he left. When I saw the team I grabbed the check off the kitchen counter and took it with me to the front door. I flung open the door and greeted the two men and one woman with a smile and a check. I said, "This is great that you stopped by, I was going to drop this by the firehouse but I see you are collecting door to door!" They looked at me like I had lost my mind! The woman member of the team said, "Are you alright ma'am? Are you feeling okay? Is there anyone here that needs medical assistance?" I stood there for a minute and then said, "I am just fine. I'm the only one home and I had just walked in from working in DC."

They told me that someone called and reported an emergency with a diabetic patient. I told them we did have a neighbor a few streets over that had been having health issues but no one here! At that moment our home phone rang. I asked the rescue team into the house and ran to answer the phone. That is when I started to put the pieces together to what was happening. The man on the phone was calling from Ray's and Evie's condo. He was with the rescue team from their area and told me that Evelyn was in grave condition and that they were taking her to the emergency room.

The local Emergency Room was closed due to a large volume of patients and they were heading to a hospital in Bethesda. I told them that I would meet them there and asked if they could please take Ray with them to the hospital because it would take me more than an hour of travel time to get to him. They agreed to transport him. They assessed that Ray was not well and decided to get both of them checked out. I thanked the team at my house and quickly explained what had happened and then showed them to the door.

I ran around gathering up some clothes and toiletries on the chance I had to spend the night in town. As if events could not get more bizarre, a call came in on my cell phone from the pharmacy in the city that we had used for over thirty years. This was a bit unusual at that time since neither Bob nor I were taking any medications. The owners, Robert and Marie, were dear friends who were more like an aunt and uncle to us, watching our children grow up and being there anytime we needed words of wisdom or advice. When I answered, it was their pharmacy tech, Virginia, calling to give me some bad news. Robert had gotten sick three days before and went into kidney failure. Virginia began to cry, she then said that Robert did not respond to treatment and passed away early that morning. Since their religious beliefs required a funeral service within twenty-four hours after death, the funeral was already scheduled to be held the next morning. No one had been called because it all happened so quickly; needless to say, I was stunned!! It had been only two weeks since I stopped by to see them. They both were fine at the time and were even planning a vacation. I thanked Virginia for calling me and told her to let us know if we could do anything for Marie and that I was dealing with a family crisis and on my way to the Emergency Room. I assured her I would be at the funeral service in the morning if possible, but it would all depend on Evelyn's condition.

I wanted to sit down and cry but knew I needed to stay focused and get to Ray and Evie. While grabbing a suit and accessories for the funeral as I was about to leave, the house phone rang again. It was the rescue squad informing me that they were changing routes because they did not think that Evie would survive the longer drive. Then I really started to panic! If she died and there wasn't family there to comfort Ray, he would fall apart and I feared he would become combative. I jumped in my car and began the race back to the city.

Once on the road I called Courtney and left a message explaining what was happening and asked her to call me as soon as possible. She was now covering the Pentagon and was attending a work dinner with members of the Joint Chiefs of Staff so her phone was off. She and I were the only ones around since Gretchen was also out of town. I called Bob in Kansas City and he said he was going to change his flight to the first one in the morning and would meet me either at the hospital or at Robert's funeral.

About twenty minutes later as I was merging onto the Beltway, I received a call from one of the doctors at the Emergency Room. To my surprise, it was Jack, one of the doctors from the Cancer Center where I had worked. He was on call for the practice and the hospital staff called him after they reviewed Evelyn's past medical records and saw the physicians from the center listed as the providers. He informed me it was really bad and to get there ASAP!!

By now I was "flying low" on the road and starting to call my family to tell them what was happening. Courtney called and said she was in her car and heading to the hospital. About ten minutes before I pulled into the hospital parking lot Jack called again and said to come straight back to the exam rooms because he did not think she had much time, in fact, she may be gone when we arrive. By some miracle Courtney and I arrived safely and at the same time. We ran past the security guards at the door and straight back to the wards. As we rounded the corner to go into the room we ran into Jack who was shaking his head. We both froze, thinking she must have died.

Jack took my hand and said, "You won't believe this, Evelyn is awake and asking for something to eat!" I didn't know whether to laugh, cry or punch Jack for making me crazy! We all walked back to her bed and there was Ray sitting in a chair holding her hand, while Evie was smiling and saying she had no idea how she got into the hospital? Courtney and I at that point looked at each other and burst out in laughter at the insanity of the last two Razzle Dazzle hours. We could not look at each other without losing our composure. It was a definite relief that Evie survived, but they had managed to turn about a dozen people's lives upside down! I was lucky that the state police did not have a warrant out for my arrest for driving like a wild woman on the Interstates.

Evie was admitted to the hospital to get her blood sugar levels stable and we took Ray to the grocery store to pick up food and then took him home. We made him dinner and got him settled for the night. It was one o'clock in the morning when I finally arrived back at my home. I initially felt I should have stayed with him but he was obviously quite nervous we were there. They both always preferred to be alone, and to be frank, the condo was so dusty I knew I would have had an allergy attack and would not be useful to anyone. I also knew that Ray would not allow me to clean the place so I decided to go home. I eventually became confident Ray would be fine and wouldn't leave the condo. We made sure to preset the coffee pot and had breakfast rolls, cereal and fruit ready for his breakfast in the morning; we definitely did not want him turning on the stove or oven. Now that Evelyn was stable, I planned to be back and take him out for lunch and to the hospital after Robert's service. To this day, we don't know who called the rescue personnel to the condo or the name of the young man that placed the 911 call to our rescue squad.

Evie was released from the hospital after two days and they managed for a few months more on their own. Her trip to the emergency room had a lasting impact on Ray and he became a regular on the phone with the 911 operators. One morning Evie awoke early, around six a.m., to find Ray and a rescue team standing at the end of her bed. She was asleep and not in any distress, but Ray had called for the paramedics because he did not think she was breathing.

The family continued attempts to get them assistance but they refused. The next step was to try to reach their primary care physician and have an intervention. We managed to find out when they were scheduled for their next visit and talked them into letting us drive them to the appointment. Of course, we had to bribe them with the offer to take them out to lunch as our treat!

While in the waiting room of the medical office, Bob was sitting next to Evie. With a concerned expression on his face he glanced over at me and nodded towards Evie's purse. Evie had opened her purse to retrieve a tissue and as she pulled it out, a wad of cash came out with it. She then quickly pushed the cash back into her purse. Bob later told me that there had to be a few thousand dollars in the bag. He was concerned that if anyone saw her in a store or public place with that much cash she could possibly be attacked for the money. Bob was concerned for our safety too!!! When we asked her later why she had so much cash in her bag she said Ray wanted her to keep the money there so it would be safe. Upon further investigation we discovered Evie was taking all the checks they received to the bank, cashing them, but not depositing any of the money into their accounts. She said with much conviction, "Ray knows the financial institutions are robbing us of our money."

After a brief stay in the waiting room Evie and Ray were called back to the exam room and Bob and I accompanied them. When the physician walked in she looked quite shocked to see Bob and I in attendance. She asked us to wait in her office as she conducted their exams. After, she met with us privately to discuss options for their care.

The doctor told us that she had asked on many visits if Ray and Evelyn had anyone she could call in case of an emergency but they denied having any family in the area. We informed her that we had been begging them to let us help and they refused. We also asked if we could get Social Services to intervene. However, we were informed that the only way we could do anything is if they fit a set of medical parameters. But, since they managed to pass all the tests we did not have any rights to intervene at this point and there was no legal recourse because we were not their children. Sadly, it would take a fall, an accident or a grave illness to change their lives and open the door to allow us to intervene.

We called Social Services and heard the same story, unless we could prove a list of problems that their hands were tied. Getting old, not eating properly and having a dirty house was not enough to force them to get help.

CHAPTER TWELVE

LET THE NURSING HOME GAMES BEGIN!

Less than three years after our 2004 feast Ray fell at their condo, Evelyn called 911 and he was taken by rescue squad to the hospital. Evelyn followed the ambulance in their car. The events of that day would begin the downward spiral we knew was inevitable. Neither of them ever stepped foot inside their home again. As Evie was standing next to Ray's bed in the Emergency Room, she experienced a diabetic incident, most likely caused by the stress. Her blood sugar fell and she passed out onto the floor hitting her face and head on the metal railings of Ray's bed. She had extensive bruising and fractured her cheek bone.

They were in the hospital for five days telling the staff that they had no family, only their elderly sisters living out of state. Ray's paranoia manifested at a new level. When he was finally alert and able to get a good look at Evelyn's injuries he went wild screaming at the staff that she had been attacked. The Social Services at the hospital were desperate to find someone that they could call to arrange rehab for Evie and nursing facilities for Ray. Apparently they had not researched the old medical files where they could have traced us by contacting the Cancer Center.

By luck, one of Jack's partners, Tim, was doing rounds at the hospital and saw their names on the patient roster board. He knew they were my aunt and uncle because he had treated my aunt for a blood disorder in the past. He walked into their room and said the look on their faces told all, they had been busted! Ray, being his frugal self, asked Tim if he was going to charge them for the visit. Tim told him he just wanted to say hello and see how they were doing. As soon as Tim left the room he went to Social Services and then called me on my cell phone. I was about to pull out of my driveway heading to a girls weekend at the Delaware beaches with some of my friends when I received the call.

Plans quickly changed and my oldest brother

James and I met an hour later at an attorney's office and filed papers to obtain an emergency guardianship. We then traveled to the hospital and met with the staff to ascertain the next move. We were informed that in their current conditions they had six months to a year to live at most and could not go back to their home. Our long term adventures in elder care were about to begin!

James and I walked into Ray's and Evie's hospital room and we were shocked to see the level of decline. Ray was so agitated that when I walked over to the side of his bed to take his hand and give him a hug he violently grabbed my arm. Fortunately, my brother was able to detach his grip before any harm was done. The social worker told us that Ray needed to go to a facility that could treat his psychological changes along with his physical medical conditions. I could not bear to place him in a psychiatric hospital. We had only two choices, a hospital in Baltimore or a skilled nursing home with a psychiatric lock down unit in Montgomery County where they lived. Fortunately the nursing home had an opening and after reviewing his medical status would accept him for treatment.

Evie had to be sent to a rehab center. We chose one that had previously treated my sister-in-law's mother. They did an amazing job getting her functioning after a fall which gave us confidence they could possibly help Evie. It wasn't a fancy place but they offered excellent care.

Ray and Evie ended up in two different facilities; over a one hour drive separated them for the first time in their married life. They were deeply in love and it broke our hearts to see them apart. But, we had no choice, they each had specific requirements and we had to take care of their emergent healthcare needs. The doctors told us the separation could prove to help them both heal, since together they declined to a dangerous level.

We only had a short window of time to get them settled into the care centers while Medicare and their secondary health insurance would cover the cost of their care. Our emergency guardianship was limited and, until we had our case heard in a court of law and permanent guardianship petitions signed, we had no access to their funds.

Court appointed attorneys were assigned to represent Ray and Evie to protect their rights and ascertain that they truly could not handle their own affairs and that we were not taking advantage of their situation. Interviews and visits were made prior to the court date. The elder attorney we hired to represent our petition and the court appointed attorneys met and agreed that the emergency guardianship should be made permanent with court supervision and annual accountings to protect all parties. The judge hearing the case approved and we officially became their legal guardians.

The legal issues ended up being the easy part, the

real challenges were just beginning. Bob and I met James and Janie at Ray's and Evie's condo to begin the job of managing their affairs and try to piece together what funds we had to work with to pay for their care. No one had walked into the apartment for a couple of weeks and we had to try to clean up the place before we started the search. What we discovered was that Evie's purse filled with money wasn't the only item filled with cash. They had stashed thousands of dollars around their condo too! We had to meticulously go through every piece of clothing, books where they had cut out hidden compartments in the pages to fit stacks of cash, drawers, kitchen and bathroom cabinets, everything!! We found financial statements and money hidden in coffee cans, the freezer and under the mattresses; we didn't dare throw out anything until we examined its contents.

Identifying the banks where they had accounts was the first priority. We then spent days traveling around the city to financial institutions armed with legal documents from the courts to prove we were their guardians and had permission to access their funds and various safety deposit boxes. Most cooperated but a few gave us a hassle even with the court orders. New accounts had to be established with our names and the funds transferred. Until we were able to locate the money and obtain access to the funds, we had to pay out of our pockets for their care beyond what insurance covered. I personally had to write a check for $10,000 to secure a room at an assisted living facility so Evie had a place to go after Medicare funds ran out and she was released from rehab. To this day we wonder if we missed finding all of their accounts. It truly was a modern day treasure hunt!

Our attorney supervised all the documentation and we hired a financial advisor to oversee their investments. We did this as much to protect ourselves as Ray and Evie. Interestingly, relatives we had never met or heard of suddenly began appearing. It's amazing how concerned people become when they think they are going to get a financial windfall.

I had one in-law relative call and yell at me because her husband did not get a picture from the White House that was a Staff Christmas gift to Evie from the Kennedy's. Evie had a number of gifts from the presidents she served over the years. As we went through the process of clearing out their property, family members informed us that all of the nieces and nephews on both sides of the family had each been told by Evie and Ray that they would leave the White House mementos to them! I told the niece it was not my decision and that she needed to call the judge!

James and I divided the rest of the duties. I paid all the bills and dealt with insurance and financial issues while James and Janie took care of getting all of their assets appraised so we had an accounting for the courts and could liquidate the property to cover the cost of their care. Together, the two healthcare facilities base fees totalled an average of $20,000 per month. We all pitched in to clean out the condo and prepare it for sale. Nonetheless, our efforts were only the first stage because the condo had to be rehabbed in order to list it for sale. Fortunately, we were able to secure a reliable contractor and realtor to work with us to get it into marketable condition.

Once Ray and Evie were placed into a safe environment, were being properly nourished and had their medications administered and monitored, they gained back strength and became stable. Ray's psychological state went back to a normal level and he once again became the lovable teddy bear we all knew and loved. We were able to move Evie to an assisted living facility and, although she missed Ray, she flourished with the social contact. We decorated her little apartment with her special treasures from their world travels and bought all new furniture. Finally, she was in a clean, safe environment and able to be a part of a community. Janie's mother was also a resident there so she had extended family living under the same roof and James and Janie were able to make frequent visits.

Evie lived for two years in the apartment and once a week we had a medical transport with an aide take her to visit Ray. The nursing home required an escort for Evelyn to visit because they did not want the liability if she fell. They had reviewed her medical records as part of their admission policy when we requested for her to be placed on their waiting list for a room. We knew eventually there would be a physical decline from the diabetes and we wanted Ray and Evie to be together in the same nursing home when the need arose.

After two years of stable health Evie's blood sugar levels began to swing wildly even with continued monitoring. The medical staff at the assisted living facility advised us to notify the nursing home that we needed to begin the plans for a move. Evie's medical issues were reaching a point beyond the care level she was being provided at that time and she needed to go to a facility that was equipped to handle the ever increasing complications of her diabetes.

By now, Ray had been moved to a regular room and had a roommate. He was totally bedridden and was only moved from the bed to a special geriatric chair. Thankfully, he was alert and enjoyed visitors and chatting with his roommate. The decision was made to place Evie across the hall in a private room so she would be close to Ray but also could have some time to herself. We found that the arrangement worked well.

With the proper care Ray survived three-and-a-half years after the fall and Evelyn four. She died one day short of six months after Ray. My dad used to tease Ray that he could not take his money with him when he died. As it turned out, Ray and Evie almost did!

After paying for other living expenses such as clothing and additional medications not covered under health insurance, plus attorney fees and pre-paying all of their funeral expenses, there was only $4,000 left when Evie died. It was as if Ray had timed how long they would live and how much money would be needed. They never had to go on any federal or state assistance programs and Ray never paid a penny to an attorney for a Will or left anyone anything. Thank God he was cheap! That enabled us to provide the best of care for them in the last years of their lives without any financial worries.

CHAPTER THIRTEEN

PLEASE CLEAN OUT YOUR HOUSE

My Mother always said, "We are victims of our own possessions." Those were wise words which none of us ever listened to and now regret as we are reaching our retirement years and are now beginning to think about downsizing. My family had a unique perspective when it came to the final stages of life because we were in the funeral business. From a very young age I witnessed families struggle, clinging together or going to war with each other over family possessions and funeral plans.

Growing up in the family business gave me a unique insight into how to comfort people while they faced the loss of their love ones and dealt with life altering events. These early life lessons prepared me for my later work endeavors as a medical administrator and gave me the skills to take on the guardianship for my aunt and uncle. I learned to cope with life's tragedies and challenges by finding the humor in the absurdity.

My dad was amazing in teaching us the art of caring for families and instilling strong administrative skills to organize and plan events from small private gatherings to large public spectacles. The oldest of eight children, he was a very spiritual person and extremely generous. At one time he seriously considered becoming a priest. Dad changed his mind when he realized he wanted a family of his own and had an interest in following his father's career path by becoming a funeral director. His examples didn't end with teaching us to run a business, he also gave back to our community. He was twice honored by the Chamber of Commerce and a local business group as the "Man of the Year" and the "Humanitarian of the Year."

My siblings and I all helped out at the funeral home, acquiring a strong work ethic by rolling up our sleeves to do whatever job needed to be completed. Some of our chores included cleaning the building, hauling flowers to the cemeteries and washing the fleet of cars. Both of my parents were opened minded, non-judgmental and encouraged us to learn new tasks and expand our skills.

The business telephone lines connected to our house. Directors are always on call twenty-four hours a day and we grew up in the days before answering services became part of the funeral business culture. As a result, we were all taught to answer the business phones. Five children and two dogs were trained to instantly become quiet when the funeral home phones rang and we were never to allow them to ring more than two times. We were versed in the proper terminology and etiquette and we followed the rules without a deviation from the protocol. My dad developed a records log we could fill out and follow to obtain the necessary information and give instructions to the caller. I actually took my first death call at the age of nine!

When we were old enough to drive my dad took us out on the road and taught us how to handle driving a limousine and a hearse. Learning to judge distances to maneuver and stop a large vehicle in a funeral procession could pose quite a challenge to a new driver. People would look a bit surprised when a five foot, two inch, sixteen year old girl would be their limo driver. But, we were very well trained and, once in the funeral procession, I proved I could handle the job. My driving claim to fame is that I can parallel park a limo and a hearse!

We were also probably the only kids in town with business suits so we looked presentable to represent the business as drivers, visitation greeters and assistants at services. My dad was very dapper and always impeccably dressed. When he first went into business with his father in the early 1940's they wore formal mourning suits. The pants had a pin stripe down the side of the leg and the jackets had tails. They also wore top hats! Fashion standards eased a bit by the 1960's and 70's and my dad always kept up with the trends. He made sure we looked professional, classic and polished in spite of our young ages.

It was actually Dad, and not my mother, who influenced my love of clothes and jewelry. Every year on my birthday starting at age three, he would take me to see his jeweler friend, the owner of a local family jewelry store and let me choose from the case filled with children's items. My mother and grandmother were convinced that they added a display case of children's watches, rings and bracelets because of my dad!

I always felt that my dad escaped all of the sadness he witnessed in his work by having diversions to enjoy. He was ahead of his time when it came to technology and eating healthy. He also was a great believer in trying cuisines from around the world. Every Friday night we went out for dinner and Dad would carefully peruse the menu and order items we had never tasted; he always tried to expose us to new tastes and textures. We dressed up, learned how to behave in a formal setting and expanded our horizons to not be afraid of trying new things.

Dad's biggest passion though was his love of cars. He became an avid collector of all types of automobiles; antiques, sports cars, and a few more "Avant Guard" vehicles that he hid from Mom! My siblings and I always laughed when one of our children or grandchildren expressed interest in cars and trucks; we knew they had inherited their PapPap's car gene!

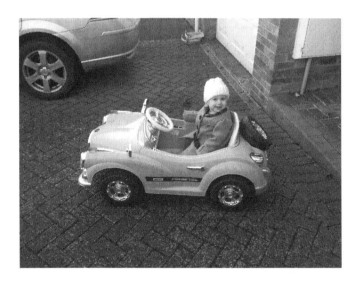

Great-granddaughter Vivien inherited PapPap's car gene.

My mom, who was much more practical and did not want to spend money on frivolous purchases, was always the last one to know when Dad bought a new toy! But for all her disapproval she too caught the car bug!

Carting around five kids in a big station wagon was not what mom had envisioned in her pursuit of becoming a career woman. In fact, Mom's first career interest was in the funeral business. One of her best friends in elementary school would take her to visit his dad's mortuary and she became fascinated by the profession. She expressed to her parents the desire to go to Mortuary School after high school. My Grandma Helen, though being a career women with the IRS and very opened minded, quickly talked Mom out of pursuing that path and instead encouraged her to get a degree in English and then consider eventually going on to Law school. How ironic that Mom would marry into a family of funeral directors! Not only was she now a part owner of a funeral home, but she also had more cars registered in her name than most women had hats or shoes!

Mom eventually put her own stamp on the car collection. One day while leafing through a magazine she spotted an advertisement for a new car being introduced by the Ford Motor Company; the Ford Mustang! My mom went crazy for the look and the design. She cut out the ad and taped it onto my dad's mirror in the bathroom with a note, "I won't complain if this is next in the fleet!" Dad surprised her by buying the first Mustang to arrive in our county, right off the truck from Detroit. It was a white convertible with red leather seats and a red pinstripe down the sides. She was ecstatic!! Funny thing though, she ended up hating the car. She had become so accustomed to driving large wagons that she was not comfortable behind the wheel. However, my three older brothers, who were in high school, were happy to take it off her hands and give her back her station wagon!

The car hobby for my dad actually turned into a sort of rehab for him too. When he was only 40 years old he had a heart attack. He was young, thin, did not smoke and did not have any of the other listed causes of being a high risk for a coronary incident. He was hit with a blood clot that caused the heart attack. He and my brothers restored a 1953 Jaguar and it did more for him then any rehab could have achieved. He looked like a member of the "Rat Pack," the famous group of Hollywood buddies led by Frank Sinatra and Dean Martin, as he tooled around town in his red Jag. Although most of his friends, after seeing him behind the wheel, started calling him Bond; after all his first name was James!

Both of my parents needed some diversion and normalcy to remind them that life is not always filled with heartache. They were tested the year my brother James, who volunteered to join the United States Army, was serving in Vietnam. My father conducted the funerals for a number of soldiers killed in the war, including my bothers best friend. Life was all too short and the social and political changes in the 1960's intensified that point. My parents faced firsthand the consequences of those times.

My mom endured the chaos and tried to remain grounded. It's funny that she was the more practical of my parents since it was her grandfather that welcomed my dad into her "Razzle Dazzle" family. Dad loved Mom's grand-dad and he would quote the "Razzle Dazzle" term to describe his own wild bunch.

My parents purchased a ski chalet in a mountain top community where the homeowners gave special names to their chalets, cottages and A-Frame retreats. Each home had a matching wooden sign post displaying their unique designation; ours was "Razzle Dazzle." When the chalet was sold I asked for the sign, a weathered reminder of my great-grandfather and Dad, now displayed at our house on the Bay.

Mom would look at all the cars and collections and loved to point out that a parents' way of "getting even with their kids" was not to downsize their lifestyles as they got older, but let the kids be stuck with the job of clearing out and disposing of their parents' treasured collections. My parents had two houses to clear out and when my dad passed away we had to track down his car collection. We suspected that he had not sold some of his many toys as he had claimed, so we contacted a few realtors to see if they had leased him garage space. Our hunch was correct! We found a limo, a sports car and two other cars he could not part with!

After working with my siblings to clean out my parents' two homes, my grandparents' apartment, Ray's and Evie's condo, and helping some of my friends pack up their parents' homes, I am ready to live like a monk! Bob's mom always laughed about her lack of treasures. Being a military family, having five boys and moving every few years, the only thing they seemed to collect was baby gear, sports equipment and toys. All kidding aside, she does have some lovely items and has asked everyone to let her know what they want and she will keep a list. Some of the family thought it was morbid but I told her she was brilliant!

Currently, ten-thousand baby boomers turn sixty-five years old each day. We are now on the brink of being the oldest generation. Some of our family and friends from our generation have begun to face life-threatening diseases and we have sadly already said goodbye to the ones who lost the fight. My advice to the world is to clean out your house, make out a will and prearrange your funeral!! Don't leave it to the courts and your kids! Take control while you still can! No, we are not going to live forever! Keep the in-laws and the outlaws from seizing control!

The reality is that your kids will probably not want all those treasures you have collected over the years. Their lifestyles are filled with technology, not fine china. I find that it sometimes skips generations and that the grandchildren want something to remember their grandparents. But don't count on it. Your kids won't want to store any of your treasured items. Let's face it, most of our kids still haven't taken all of their stuff out of our basements after "they" left home.

Looking back, we were lucky to have the resources to care for Ray and Evelyn. It was not possible for us to take care of them ourselves. As much work and stress as this was on us to oversee their care, we had it easy compared to the millions who struggle every day trying to cope with the physical care of elderly family members. Most rarely have a break from their daily responsibilities, and it often leads to caregiver burnout. These selfless individuals are our heroes.

I witnessed firsthand family care giving when Sally, who is an only child, was faced with taking care of her mother Elizabeth (or as I called her, Miss Elizabeth) in the final days of her life. Sally had promised her mother that she would care for her at home which is where Miss Elizabeth wanted to die. It became a family affair, Sally's husband Jay and their daughters, all pitched in to help as did many of Sally's friends. The last few days we all took turns spending the night with Sally and Jay since someone had to be awake 24/7 to keep watch.

We worked in shifts attending to Miss Elizabeth's care, then, one by one we would collapse on a bed or couch, wherever there was a space, to try to catch a few winks. One morning we awoke to find the three of us, me, Jay and Sally, in that order, had fallen asleep laying across the same bed side by side. Jay rolled over to see two women lying next to him and said, "If this had only happened forty years ago." In our utter exhaustion we could only lie there laughing hysterically at the outrageous sight that only true friends would find so humorous.

With little sleep we were all a bit punchy towards the end. But in true "Sally and Dianne fashion" we decided to be prepared and make sure all the arrangements were made for the funeral. They had prearrangements set with a local funeral home but they had not picked out an urn for Miss Elizabeth's ashes which were to rest beside Sally's dad at Arlington National Cemetery. I called down to Arlington to ask what the requirements were for size and material. The woman on the other end of the phone, with a heavy southern drawl, gave me the dimensions then said, "Well honey, anything y'all desire, why you can even use a coffee can if she had a special brand! Just be sure to use a lid!" I was cracking up laughing when I got off the phone!

With that bit of knowledge, Sally and I decided that Miss Elizabeth, who was a long time member of the Washington Glass Club, was going out in style! I did make a midnight phone call to my funeral director brother one night when we could not sleep to get his advice. He gave us his opinion then told us to go to bed and stop making nocturnal phone calls! We stayed up and searched through the china cabinets filled with Miss Elizabeth's treasured collection but could not find the right piece. After Miss Elizabeth passed away, Sally, me, Sally's best friend from childhood, and her mom's oldest and newest best girlfriends, took a trip to a local neighborhood that had a half dozen antique shops to find the perfect glass vessel. As the five ladies on a mission walked into the first shop and scanned the contents, a collective "that's it" rang out!

On the top shelf of a large hutch was the perfect Bristol blue glass urn with delicate flowers hand painted on one side, and it had a beautiful lid! It was the perfect resting place for a proper Southern lady. Sally said she knew her mom was looking down on us from heaven and proclaiming her favorite hymnal phrase which she quoted throughout her life, "It is well with my soul."

Sadly, most of the issues we had to deal with concerning Ray's and Evie's care, could have been avoided if Ray had not been so stubborn and agreed to assistance while they could still be a part of the decision making process. If they made the proper choices earlier they may have survived longer and had a better quality of life. Also, it would have been their choice as to whom to leave their prized possessions and they may have been able to stay together rather than being forced to be apart by circumstances.

Because there wasn't a will or any directives, the courts dictated what had to be done with their property and funds. The irony is that for all their efforts to protect their privacy and not allow anyone access to their personal affairs, their lives became an open book discussed in a public court of law. This is not a route I would recommend to any family; which takes me back to Barbara and Mel.

Barbara and Mel were both extremely organized and efficient planners. When Mel died he left explicit directions for his funeral, including choosing the caterer and the menu for the luncheon after the funeral service. Liz and Anne were able to celebrate their dad's life and he took care of and protected them to the end.

Barbara was the last survivor of our five special visitors. She lived almost ten years from Thanksgiving Day 2004. She still loved to chat with anyone within earshot. Unfortunately, she declined to a place where she could no longer speak a word of French, her adopted second language which she loved, and she had moments of confusion and asked for Mel every day. Liz said she had peace in her final days and her death was as sweet and precious as Barbara was in life. The nursing home hosted a Valentines party for the residents and Barbara participated in the fun. She ate, sang and socialized. After the festivities ended her minister dropped by for a visit; they sang Amazing Grace and read from the scriptures together. Barbara had truly enjoyed the day. She asked to be helped from her wheelchair into her bed so she could take a nap. With a big smile on her face she fell asleep and never awoke. She had gone on to be with Melvin, her Valentine.

EPILOGUE

Years later we look back on the Thanksgiving of 2004 with fond memories, amusement and melancholy. That day was filled with first and last moments. It would be the one and only time that any of these lovely souls would be with us in our home and the last time the two couples and Shirley ever saw each other. It truly was a First and Last Thanksgiving! Even with the sad passing of these lives we have also been filled and blessed with new family members and another generation being born.

Courtney and Gretchen sold their home in 2007 when Gretchen decided to head to the United Kingdom to work on a second Master's Degree and begin studies towards a Doctorate. She met a wonderful British gentleman, Matthew, who was studying medicine. They fell in love and decided to be married in London where they met. My planning skills took on a new challenge as we hosted a wedding in England and merged the wedding traditions and customs of two nations into one ceremony. Two years later our adorable little granddaughter, Vivien was born. Though not celebrated in the United Kingdom, we traveled over to celebrate her first Thanksgiving and cook a Turkey in their tiny London flat, in a kitchen the size of our walk-in closet! It was a scene playing over again for Vivien just like her mommy's first Thanksgiving thirty-five years before. It was wonderful!!!! Matthew is now a physician, a practicing Psychiatrist (every family needs one), and Gretchen heads the English Department at an all boy's prep school. Bob and I are racking up the frequent flyer miles as we "cross the pond" every few months for precious time together.

Courtney bought a restored historic townhouse a block from where my mother grew up in a gentrified section of Washington, D.C. Her career continued to grow covering politics and national security. She has traveled the world dozens of times covering stories and reporting from the Far East, Europe, South America, Africa and the Middle East, including thirty visits to the front lines in Iraq and Afghanistan. She also met the love of her life, Eric, a decorated Lieutenant Colonel and public affairs officer for the

Marine Corps. He entered our family with an added bonus, his two sons from his first marriage, Eric Ray and Ethan. Eric and the boys think I make the best turkey and stuffing they have ever tasted. We are always so happy when Eric Ray, now serving in the United States Air Force, and Ethan, just finishing school, are able to join us for celebrations and allow us to indulge them with grandparent love. Six months after their wedding, Courtney announced they were expecting their first baby, actually, first and second babies, twins, and both boys, Ryan and Jackson. The twins call their older brothers "Big Brother Eric" and "Big Brother Ethan." All four boys, big and small, embrace the times they can be together.

In addition to taking care of our elders we are on call as grandparent baby-sitters in the United States and in England. You could say we are official card carrying members of the sandwich generation, plus one; another generation to love and cherish, and yes, we are still scraping food off the floor!

Bob and I decided to document how to cook my Mom's turkey, stuffing and soup so it can be shared and enjoyed for future generations, one Thanksgiving at a time. As we prepared each stage of the meal, Bob took notes and photos recording the recipes and we added family traditions and hints for making a feast.

Ironically, last year I broke a bone in my right

foot when the sole of my shoe became caught in an expansion joint on our driveway as I was putting the trash cans into the garage. I was so fortunate that it was the only injury. I lost my balance and could not get my foot out of the shoe quick enough to prevent the fall. The calamity was so bizarre to me that I started to laugh out loud. It must have relaxed me when I hit the pavement because I didn't suffer any additional injury. Just like Evie, I was in a walking boot, but it only slowed me down for a few days; I was determined to keep on moving and driving.

Two of my girlfriends have also broken a foot or an ankle! One was walking her daughter's large dog and he wrapped the leash around her leg throwing her to the ground breaking her ankle. The other friend was on vacation with her family and forced to run down a hill to catch her grandson who had let go of her hand thinking it was funny to be naughty. We commiserate that the kids are all out to get us!

With all the jokes made about getting older and the challenges being faced by all families, age can come with clarity and wisdom, teaching us what truly matters. Through all the stages, keeping a strong sense of humor and our dignity is probably the best way to survive and enjoy life, as the caregiver or the receiver of care. This same attitude is one to remember to survive family holidays too!

This past Thanksgiving continued the trend; the table settings and flower arrangements designed for royalty, thirteen for dinner, including two, two year olds (we are still supervising loved one's going up and down the stairs), a few last minute guests, as usual, and way too many desserts!

Family and friends at the Bay House, all a bit more worn and faded, sharing a meal of comfort food, finding the time to pause from the Razzle Dazzle challenges of life to rejoice and celebrate. The spirits of our five special guests are in our hearts as we give thanks for the love and the memories. Family traditions passed down through the generations weaving the threads that hold us together, linking us from the past and into the future.

Wishing you all the best as you celebrate your holidays, through the laughter, the tears, the burnt rolls and the spilled dips, Cheers!

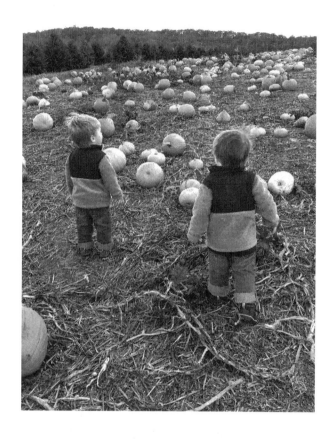

Another generation, another holiday season; Grandsons Ryan
and Jackson look for the perfect pumpkin.

APPENDIX

DIANNE'S FALL HARVEST

APPLE CAKE RECIPE

Fall Harvest Apple Cake Recipe

3 Eggs

2 Cups of Sugar

1 Cup Canola Oil

1 Teaspoon Vanilla

2 Cups Baking Flour (All-Purpose Flour or Gluten Free Flour can also be used)

2 Teaspoons Cinnamon

1 Teaspoon Baking Soda

½ Teaspoon Salt

4 Cups Cored, Pared and Sliced Baking Apples, but do not slice too thin! (4 large or 5 medium)

Optional; 1 Cup Chopped Nuts, Walnuts or Pecans

Note: I recommend using a sturdy baking apple that will keep its texture and not become mushy. My preferred varieties are Braeburn, Honeycrisp, Pink Lady, McIntosh, Gala or Fuji apples. Most are available in local markets. If the apples have a sweeter taste you can cut back on the sugar to 1 1/2 cups or a lesser amount as desired, but don't use less than 1 cup. White granulated is preferred so as to not alter the texture of the cake.

Preheat the oven to 350 degrees. Prepare a 13x9x2 baking dish by rubbing a thin coat of butter, canola oil or your preferred baking product over the bottom and sides to prevent the cake from sticking while serving. The baking dish will also serve as the serving dish.

Spread the apple slices over the bottom of the prepared baking dish to fully cover. Beat the eggs with a hand mixer until they whip into a thick blend that has a light froth on top. Pour the sugar and oil into the eggs with the mixer on medium speed, mix well scraping the sides of the mixing bowl with a spatula. Once well combined add the vanilla and mix to blend.

In a separate bowl, stir together the flour, cinnamon, baking soda and salt to blend the dry ingredients; in small portions add the dry blend into the egg mixture, this will make the mixing easier; beat until the texture of this batter is very thick. Stir in the nuts if adding to the recipe.

Pour the batter over the apples, spreading to cover the entire layer of fruit. As noted, the batter will be thick and will sink to the bottom of the dish surrounding the apple slices.

Bake at 350 degrees for one hour. The cake will rise a bit and most likely will have some cracks across the smooth top when fully baked. Remove from the oven and cool in the baking dish on a wire rack. The cake should be at room temperature or chilled in the refrigerator before icing.

Cream Cheese Icing Recipe

1, 8oz Block of Cream Cheese

¼ Cup Unsalted Butter (1/2 Stick)

1 to 2 Cups of Powdered Sugar

1 Lemon

Soften 1, 8 oz. block of cream cheese to room temperature. Beat with mixer until fluffy. Beat in ¼ cup (1/2 stick) unsalted melted butter until well blended; many cream cheese icing recipes call for up to 2 cups of powdered sugar and one teaspoon of lemon juice. I recommend adding only ½ to 1 cup of powdered sugar and a minimum of four teaspoons of lemon juice. I prefer to add the juice of one fresh lemon. I add these ingredients a small amount at a time, tasting between additions to adjust the sweetness and tartness of the icing. The icing will be smooth and creamy with this method. Increased amounts of sugar will make it fluffier; additional lemon juice will make it creamier.

Spread over the cooled cake and refrigerate to keep fresh. This cake can be made up to one week in advance or frozen for up to two months. The cake texture is best if served at room temperature. Makes 12-15 servings.

We serve this cake every Thanksgiving using fresh local apples from the fall harvest! Enjoy!!

ABOUT THE AUTHOR

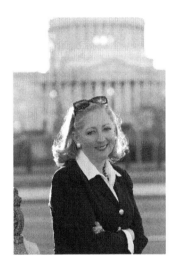

Dianne Kube, a special events and political consultant, has been on the front lines of presidential campaigns and is no stranger to Capitol Hill. Prior to her current role, with an extensive background in medical administration, Dianne advanced in her career over numerous years to eventually become the Chief Administrative Officer of a grassroots organization representing community-based cancer centers and their patients across the United States. She and a team of medical oncology professionals worked directly with Congressional Members of both political parties to develop policy changes for the Medicare Modernization Act (MMA), with the goal of protecting the quality and affordability of cancer care for all patients. Dianne has authored briefings, presentations and speeches as well as given testimony before state and federal legislatures on various healthcare policy issues. Her work also led to participation in the international healthcare arena when she was asked to join a Congressional Delegation traveling to Eastern Europe to ascertain the continued healthcare needs of citizens affected by the fallout from the Chernobyl Nuclear Power Plant Accident, for the 20th anniversary of the occurrence. Dianne has also been a sought after speaker at numerous academic, legislative and medical industry forums in the United States and in Europe. She is the mother of two accomplished daughters, the mother-in-law to two equally-accomplished sons-in-law, and enjoys every opportunity available to spend time with her five grandchildren. When not working or traveling she and her husband enjoy a full life living on the Chesapeake Bay.

Register This Book and Receive Free Updates & Dianne's Favorite Recipe

To get updates to this book and access a FREE download of Dianne's Recipe visit

www.FirstandLastThanksgiving.com

69171295R00086

Made in the USA
Lexington, KY
26 October 2017